TEACHING
THE GIFTED/LEARNING
DISABLED CHILD

Paul R. Daniels

The Johns Hopkins University

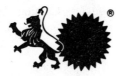

AN ASPEN PUBLICATION®
Aspen Systems Corporation
Rockville, Maryland
London
1983

Library of Congress Cataloging in Publication Data

Daniels, Paul R.
Teaching the gifted/learning disabled child.

Includes index and bibliographies.
1. Exceptional children—Education. 2. Gifted
children—Education. 3. Learning disabilities.
I. Title.
LC3965.D26   1983   371.95′6   82-22775
ISBN: 0-89443-928-6

Publisher: John Marozsan
Editorial Director: R. Curtis Whitsel
Managing Editor: Margot Raphael
Editorial Services: Eileen Higgins
Printing and Manufacturing: Debbie Collins

Library of Congress Catalog Card Number: 82-22775
ISBN: 0-89443-928-6

Printed in the United States of America

1 2 3 4 5

Table of Contents

Foreword

This book grew out of the personal experiences of the author. For 19 years I worked with children from all over the English-speaking world who had severe reading and learning disabilities. There always was a group of children who were unsuccessful in school and usually in certain aspects of their lives, and yet had more "native intelligence" than most people. Often their giftedness was measurable and was uncovered by the astute perceptions of well-trained clinicians.

After working with them and the other average and above-average children, it became evident that although these gifted young people had academic problems sometimes similar to the others, they also were different. These experiences coalesced into a set of personal concepts about gifted/learning disabled children.

Throughout those 19 years, in selected situations, the procedures that grew from these personal experiences were tried and in most cases found to be advantageous.

However, as the goals and needs of the country changed, the gifted children with learning difficulties were lost to sight and finally "disappeared." In most school systems today, it seems that they do not even exist. Yet, they do exist, though they go unrecognized. My hope is that concerned educators and parents in true justice to other human beings will accept the recognition of these children and attempt to meet their needs.

There is no attempt to make this book a scholarly work. In fact, so little is really known or understood about these children that in all probability a scholarly work could not be developed. This book is pragmatic in nature, deliberately so. The ideas, procedures, suggestions, etc., grow out of practice, not research. Therefore, they should be used that way. To readers: try things, become your own authority, and learn from the children and your experiences with them.

I hope I did.

Paul R. Daniels, Ed.D.
January 1983

Preface

There exists in the school-age population a group of students who appear to be a contradiction in terms. These are children who can legitimately be called gifted and yet at the same time be labelled learning disabled. It appears that this group has gone undetected and because of this has not received appropriate or necessary services.

The basic problem often stems from two fundamental but very subjective decisions derived from inadequate data:

1. Children who have demonstrated reading problems from their initial entrance into school may never have had their basic intelligence measured, since failure to achieve tends to be equated with average or low intellectual ability.
2. Children who have been making adequate progress—scores at or near grade level on standardized tests—do not demonstrate the need for referral. Some of these children essentially mask their disability because of their innate capacity.

Certain specific factors compound the program for gifted/learning disabled children. First, it is evident from the National Assessment of Educational Progress that schools are doing a poor job of developing critical thinking. This is an area in which gifted children should be outstanding. Disabilities in this area are highlighted in poor comprehension abilities—and disability in comprehension is under the law, a learning disability (P.L. 94-142). Yet few, if any, of these disabled children are receiving services in learning disability programs. The cause of this oversight is rather evident: the diagnostic testing for comprehension difficulties is meager at best.

Second, placement in a learning disability program requires that a severe discrepancy be determined. Severe discrepancy in terms of comprehension seldom is defined on the basis of potential. In most cases the discrepancy is between achievement and grade level. As noted, many gifted/learning disabled children are making adequate progress in light of the grade-level base line. Many of these perform adequately in literal comprehension and are considered nonhandicapped. This label surely could not be accepted if true potential for abstract thinking and/or creativity was used as the base line.

This text has been developed to help teachers, administrators, and parents better recognize and prepare for these most neglected of learning disabled children.

Acknowledgments

To the Spencer Foundation, whose support made research about gifted learning disabled children possible and stimulated an interest in their welfare.

To Mrs. Deborah Loomis, who worked so hard and well on preparing the manuscript and who cheerfully retyped materials to reflect needed changes.

To my wife, Madelyn, who encouraged me and patiently accepted my lapses in memory and distractibility.

To those bright learning disabled children I have known since 1950, who taught me so much, who sharpened my appreciations, and who fostered my humility about really understanding human beings.

To all others who taught me and from whom I have learned.

To all of the above, with my grateful thanks and appreciation, I dedicate this book.

Part I

Recognition and Diagnosis Unit

Who are they? What do they look like? How can they be found?

This unit concerns the characteristics of gifted/learning disabled children, and diagnostic procedures to identify them. Difficulties in these areas are pointed out and suggestions for actions outlined.

Chapter 1

The Population

This book deals with the instruction of those in the school-age population who fit into two categories of exceptionality at one time. To many nonprofessionals, the categories are antithetical. To many professionals in psychology and education, they are an enigma. To many families, they are a disaster.

The children find themselves puzzled by inklings of defectiveness and tormented by demands they are told they should be able to meet and yet cannot. These children are the gifted/learning disabled.

Of a large group of children with severe reading and learning problems, more than 4 percent can be identified as gifted on either a verbal or performance measure of intelligence. This figure is very close to the percentage accepted by educators of gifted children in the regular population.

This book does not and could not deal with all aspects of giftedness. It centers on children with two and, to some degree, three attributes of giftedness.

The official definition of giftedness is by Marland (1972):

Children capable of high performance include those with demonstrated achievement and/or potential ability in any of the following areas, singly or in combination:

1. general intellectual ability;
2. specific academic aptitude;
3. creative or productive thinking;
4. leadership ability;
5. visual and performing arts;
6. psychomotor ability. (p. 2)

The major focus of interest is on children who demonstrate (1) general intellectual ability, (2) creative or productive thinking, and, to a lesser degree, (3) specific

3

academic aptitude. The three other categories of giftedness undoubtedly are valid but are beyond the scope of this work.

The other exceptionality that differentiates these children is a learning disability. It must be understood clearly that no attempt is made here to give a final definition of learning disabilities. Learning disorders, learning problems, etc., are subsumed under learning disabilities. The interest is in the bright child who seems unable to achieve academically to the degree that the term giftedness might imply.

The official definition of learning disabilities (P.L. 94-142) states:

"Specific learning disability" means a disorder in one or more of the basic psychological processes involved in understanding or in using language, spoken or written, which may manifest itself in an imperfect ability to listen, think, speak, read, write, spell, or do mathematical calculations. The term includes such conditions as perceptual handicaps, brain injury, minimal brain dysfunction, dyslexia, and developmental aphasia. The term does not include children who have learning problems which are primarily the result of visual, hearing, or motor handicaps, of mental retardation, of emotional disturbance, or of environmental, cultural, or economic disadvantage.

SUBGROUPS OF GIFTED CHILDREN

Viewed from the achievement standpoint, gifted children can fit into four major categories:

1. gifted, with no learning, reading, or language disability
2. gifted, with no learning, reading, or language disability but not performing at their potential academic level
3. gifted, with a learning disability, but functioning at grade level
4. gifted, with a learning disability, but not succeeding either at grade level or level of academic potential.

Gifted Achievers

The gifted children who are successful in their schooling seem to be relatively few in number. Little in this book is directed toward them and no major thrust into this area of gifted education is implied.

Gifted Nonachievers

Some children with high intellectual possibilities are not demonstrating this potential in academic areas. They suffer not from learning or reading disabilities but rather from programmatic retardation or programmatic difficulties. They often are in programs based on grade-level goals and objectives that preclude much academic progress beyond the grade. Even in schools where such children are recognized as having above-average potential, efforts such as those called enrichment programs are devised that limit progress so that instructional and management problems are not created in the following year's activities.

Analysis of this procedure would reveal that as children progress through the grades, they are in effect becoming more retarded academically. Goals that could be reached obviously become greater and greater as the students mature but the difference between "what might have been" and "what is" grows more pronounced since an arbitrary upper limit has been placed on their progress.

This problem, once again, is not the major focus of this text although use of some of the suggested elements of classroom management and instructional procedures could reduce both specific programmatic retardation and the number of children suffering from it.

Gifted Pseudoachievers

Another subgroup is possibly the least recognized of the population: those who are genuinely gifted but also are genuinely learning disabled. They go unrecognized fundamentally because their giftedness masks the disability.

In school systems where achievement is based on standardized test scores, with grade-level placement being the sought-after goal, these children are unnoticed. Such systems usually refer them for help or recognized problems only if they make inferior grade-level scores on those tests. Since these children tend to operate at or close to grade level, their needs in effect go unrecognized. It would be of real interest and value if the percentage of these children could be discovered.

They are truly retarded in achievement if a measure of potential is used to determine retardation; many of them are truly disabled, especially in the basic process skills. Again, it appears that this disability and resulting real retardation often go totally undetected or are discerned so late in the students' academic career that effective remediation is limited.

Attention needs to be given in assessment and diagnostic procedures to the discovery of these children so that proper remediation can be provided as early as possible.

Gifted/Learning Disabled

In contrast to the gifted pseudoachievers, another group of children is identified as gifted yet is recognized as having learning disabilities. In contrast to the achieving learning disabled pupils, these fail to succeed. Any attempt to explain why these two groups exist would be pure conjecture and of little immediate practical value.

From the beginning of formal academic instruction, most of these children have been recognized as having learning problems but unfortunately, because of such early identification, many have not been discerned as gifted. Because of the specific traits listed in the next chapter, educators tend to give little or no thought to a detailed evaluation. In fact most schools feel they have a remedial system already in place to meet these needs. Therefore, in a real sense it is not a matter of a system's indifference or neglect; rather, it is a failure to investigate all the dimensions of the children's being. (See Chapter 4 on early identification of these pupils.)

Once again, unfortunately, students can be placed in a remedial program that does not meet their intellectual needs and that further exacerbates their problems. In many cases, feelings of defectiveness and despair are the end product of such well-intentioned but unsuitable programs.

It should be evident that educational neglect of the gifted/learning disabled has prevented a large number of individuals from making their contributions to society and the world. The potential of the very intelligent to perceive solutions or answers to pressing problems has always been accepted. Their ability to engage in divergent thinking that recognizes more and varied solutions to problems has not always been appreciated, yet it has been recognized that they often are the source of progress.

Horror stories of neglect and insensitivity could be recounted but they only help increase sensitivity to the concept that gifted/learning disabled children exist. This text is intended to heighten such sensitivity and provide diagnostic and prescriptive procedures to facilitate the recognition and appropriate educational treatment for these pupils.

SUMMARY

Four different types of gifted children appear to be identifiable. Of the four, the pseudoachiever and the gifted/learning disabled child are the focus of this book. True identification of these two types often is neglected because of the nature of their problems. The pseudoachievers are missed because they do not appear as failures. Their scores on achievement tests tend to approach the mean of the grade, so no alert is sounded. The gifted/learning disabled usually demonstrate their disabilities early in school and the dysfunction is treated, often as an isolated factor. When such a program is inaugurated, the giftedness often goes undetected.

Both groups suffer because of the lack of recognition of the polarity of their exceptionalities. Prescriptive practices therefore are often less than appropriate. The true nature of these children is undetected and, in far too many instances, the end product is harm rather than good.

Sadly, this harm develops in most cases out of concern that is genuine. The limitations in this concern brought about by the failure to recognize both giftedness and disability are the elements that schools and parents must recognize.

REFERENCES

Marland, S.E. *Education of the Gifted and Talented* (Vol. 1). Report to the Congress of the United States by the U.S. Commissioner of Education. Washington, D.C.: U.S. Government Printing Office, 1972.

Public Law 94-142, the *Education for All Handicapped Children Act of 1975*, Sec. 620(b)(4)(A), 89 Stat. 794.

Chapter 2

Characteristics and Traits

Gifted/learning disabled children demonstrate the same basic identifying dysfunctional characteristics as their less problematic peers. Difficulty with time concepts, the need for multisensory stimulation for word learning, quick changes of interest, etc., can be discerned in both groups. Too frequently these basic traits go unnoticed or undetected because intensive observation or diagnosis is not carried out. One reason for this oversight is that the recognition of giftedness overshadows the recognition of the learning disability.

However, gifted/learning disabled children demonstrate four major traits that are not characteristic of gifted children as a whole. They involve vocabulary, speed of reaction, flexibility, and adaptability. Usually these traits are found to be quite marked if a serious attempt is made to observe them. All four traits may not appear in each child but a constellation of at least three is to be expected.

VOCABULARY

Gifted/learning disabled children usually appear to do better than average on vocabulary tests. A grade level or scaled score of this ability seldom indicates the problem. These pupils often demonstrate impressive (listening and reading) and expressive (speaking and writing) deficits in vocabulary. These do not appear as a type of dysphasia but rather as a noticeable failure to read on an obviously higher or more sophisticated level. In many instances, the children's conversations are stilted and their speaking and writing reflect little creativity of expression. During listening activities, they do not seem to appreciate verbal humor, puns, plays on words, sarcasm, jargon, etc. These same tendencies also can be noted in their approaches to printed materials. The vocabulary they use and understand tends to be flat.

These pupils seem to have no definitive difficulty in acquiring vocabulary. In most cases, they perform better than their chronological peers. Their problems are seen more clearly in semantic variation. In conventional reading programs they tend to learn the vocabulary if it is adapted to their needs. Often, however, that is the only vocabulary they learn. This same tendency is apparent in a conventional vocabulary program to which they are exposed. Possibly because of their problems, they tend not to engage in activities that would broaden their language base. They usually do not read widely for pleasure since it is not enjoyable. They may focus on one intense interest and miss the language growth inherent in appreciating a wide area of subjects.

Vocabulary analyses of these students often yield profiles that geometrically resemble an obelisk, rather tall but narrow, with their test scores representing the height. By contrast, vocabulary development in most nondisabled gifted children resembles an isosceles triangle. The height to the apex still is apparent in tests but the broad base is perceived only through observation. The figures picture well the characteristics of the two groups: the vocabularies of gifted/learning disabled children tend to be narrow and unstable while those of their nondisabled peers have strong, sturdy, supportive language structures, demonstrated in their appreciation of semantic variation and language creativity.

SPEED OF REACTION

Many gifted/learning disabled children tend to be plodding in their behavior in many areas, especially academic ones. Their speed of reaction once again is not that of a neurologically damaged child; rather, it tends to be stylized or ponderous. At times, it appears that they are giving too much thought to behavior that really ought to be nearly automatic. They always seem to need to think things through.

It may well be that they feel this tendency is a useful defense mechanism. Most of them have failed in their own eyes and in the eyes of their parents and teachers so it is possible that this apparent slowness of reaction is a technique to keep failure at a minimum by attempting to guarantee success. Unfortunately, this tendency to ponder often guarantees more failure, especially in academic areas where speed of reaction can pay more dividends than accuracy. This is especially true in most instructional settings. The child who is slow often is criticized by the group and the teacher and is regarded as a hindrance or pest. Gifted/learning disabled children do not need more guilt or hurt than they already have. This problem is especially acute for children whose teachers and peers know they are gifted.

This stylized, pondering behavior is devastating in another crucial area—standardized test taking. Since nearly all standardized tests are timed, children who work slowly tend to be penalized. Few tests have accuracy scores (the ratio of items correct to items attempted); therefore, pupils who can move through a test rapidly tend to encounter more items for which they know the answer or can make a good guess. Gifted/learning disabled children have a tendency to ponder over the test item by item so that in an allotted time they encounter fewer items than their nonhandicapped peers and thus have the opportunity for fewer correct responses. Their overall scores surely do not reflect their capabilities in many cases. Once again, this trait generates despair and reinforces more negative feelings.

FLEXIBILITY

Highly intelligent people usually are expected to be flexible in their approaches to life situations. Gifted/learning disabled children often fail to demonstrate such flexibility. They tend to learn a technique or develop a procedure and cling to it. They find it very difficult to accept the concept that another technique or procedure is better or more appropriate to deal with a problem. For many of these children the simple suggestion that there are a number of ways to approach a task is unnerving. A kind of panic sets in, accompanied by a "what's-the-use" attitude. It is almost as if flexibility destroys their structured world and leaves only chaos, which they cannot handle.

Rules, regulations, mastered systems, etc., tend to supply these students with a perceived structure. Once structure is gone, terror replaces it. This characteristic seems to be a factor in most learning disabled children; it does not appear to be a problem for the gifted. In this respect, many gifted children thrive on the opportunity to develop flexibility, but gifted/learning disabled ones appear not to do so.

ADAPTABILITY

Most normal and above-average children can face tasks or situations and adapt their behavior in ways that are appropriate to the demands. Gifted/learning disabled children often find it extremely difficult to give up a technique or procedure that they have been using. When faced with a need to adapt, they may resort to rigidity. This lack of adaptability produces an air of hopelessness. The concept that things and situations change and, therefore, the students themselves must, can be overwhelming. These very bright children tend to see themselves as pawns in the hands of fate, unable to control their destinies. This marionette quality is reflected in their complaints of always being maneuvered by siblings, parents, classmates, and teachers. To many of these children, life is a game that they must play in which the rules are constantly changing. They see this social instability as preventing progress.

This lack of adaptability in fact may be the basic reason why gifted/learning disabled children often are charged with being unmotivated. In truth, they may have developed an attitude of "What does it matter? I can't do anything about it anyway." This type of despair could well arise when they cannot adapt to changing circumstances and demands. Some bankers and stockbrokers in the Great Depression committed suicide, while others adapted to their circumstances and regained their fortunes. Gifted/learning disabled children often are at the mercies of their own routines.

In this population is another group that is not identified as gifted because of learning disabilities. These children often are identified early in their schooling and are provided with "appropriate service"—remedial instruction. In many instances the disabilities are so evident that no attempt is made to measure intellectual potential, and the giftedness goes undiscovered.

The damaging factors in such situations lie in the lack of stimulation provided to the children. Placed in a regimented, sterile skills development program, their potential is prevented from blossoming. The rigidity of these programs plays into the pupils' lack of flexibility and adaptability and reinforces them as appropriate behaviors. The value and usefulness of basic high intelligence never are brought to bear for the good of the children or society.

The well-intentioned early identification of learning disabilities may very well mean that large numbers of gifted/learning disabled children are unidentified. A valid way to measure intellectual potential could prevent this.

EMOTIONAL ASPECTS

Most gifted/learning disabled children, even those who have gone undetected, have suffered emotional trauma of some type. The strongest blows usually are to their egos. They suffer a loss of self-esteem, self-worth, confidence, and initiative. In light of these circumstances it is reasonable to expect defense mechanisms to develop. These students tend to use three of these rather regularly: denial, projection, and rationalization. It is interesting to note that parents often use these mechanisms, too.

Denial

Many of these children simply refuse to accept the fact that they have problems, whether the problem is as broad as underachieving in all academic areas or as narrow as not knowing how to write certain words. At times the teacher, and in some instances the parents, feel like throttling the children because their denials seem so irrational. The denials may even carry over into career goals. Some children simply refuse to accept the fact that certain careers require specific academic skills.

One totally illiterate, very bright 14-year-old decided he would become a physician like his father. The fact that he said he would was enough. Some day, no matter what his abilities, he would be a doctor. It must be noted that these statements at the time were reassuring enough to himself that he could go on. His acceptance of reality could have caused his world to collapse at that time. However, as understanding grew and counseling was provided, a career was decided upon, not without considerable effort. Parents follow the same behavior in the belief or hope that eventually things will work out. When both segments of the family agree in this deception, remediation is difficult.

Projection

Whenever denial is put aside, projection nearly always is used in its place. Projection is a technique for placing blame elsewhere. The children blame parts of themselves, as if those parts were independent: "It's that dumb brain of mine," or, "My rotten fingers did it wrong." Some learning disabled children use this mechanism but it also is quite common in gifted nonachieving ones.

Parents use projection in another way. They tend to blame a past learning experience: "There were no problems until my child was in third grade," or, "in X's room." Investigation usually discloses that problems existed before the situation arose. Many parents cannot accept their child's handicap or fear that they may be responsible for it. In some cases, this projection includes the child. Parents can accept the term "learning disabled" or "dyslexic" but not "emotionally disturbed." In essence, the former labels mean that the problem is in the child, while the latter might put the family or parents in a bad light. Unfortunately, in some cases, the parents' projections become the children's rationalizations.

Rationalization

Rationalization is finding excuses. The most intense form of rationalization used by gifted/learning disabled children tends to be nontrying. Not trying allows a child to say, "I could have done it, but I didn't try," or, "If I try, I can do it." The self-deception can be very soothing. In teaching situations, the emotional reactions engendered by this rationalization become profound. Learning requires trying and trying involves failures. The full circle of the adjustment difficulties sparkles and crackles like a faulty electrical circuit. And as in that faulty circuit, progress is halted or interrupted.

These mechanisms often are demonstrated in a single behavior. The children tend to be passively aggressive. They get their way by a type of nonviolent behavior or passivity. In some instances, they refuse to respond to questions, talk, or look at the teacher. They put the instructor in a rather hopeless position. The pupils cannot be struck or forced to talk. In too many cases, they get their way. They avoid the issue or do not deal with the problem.

For a teacher, this can be a most trying experience. It cannot be dealt with using nondirective techniques since these play into the problems. Instructors need to be trained as educational therapists if they are to cope with such situations. (For more on this issue, see Chapter 14, on the teacher as learning therapist.)

One of the truly profound decisions that must be made about a program for gifted/learning disabled children has its origin in the characteristics already discussed. Must the child receive psychotherapy before educational progress can be made? The only answer appears to be pragmatic. If in four or five months the educational program seems to be solving the problem, it should be continued; if academic success has not resulted, appropriate psychotherapy should be provided. Abrams (1980) provides a thorough discussion of the emotional aspects of learning disorders.

SUMMARY

When it becomes necessary to evaluate a child who on valid evaluation measures such as the Stanford-Binet or the Wechsler Intelligence Scale for Children (WISC), for example, demonstrates a superior intelligence yet is academically lacking in achievement or is minimally successful, it must be recognized that positive results in reading and learning depend on more than intelligence. There seem to be four discernible attributes that these children are missing:

1. They lack vocabulary sophistication and appreciation.
2. They lack speed of reaction, especially in language areas.
3. They tend to be rigid and nonflexible in their approaches to problems.
4. They find it difficult to react to situations that differ from their perceived routines.

An educator who notices an intellectually endowed pupil who is academically unsuccessful and who demonstrates three of those traits probably has discovered a gifted child who is learning disabled. It is possible that one of the reasons these children have been missed for so many years is that they do not exhibit all the classic symptoms of reading and learning disability discussed in the literature. Their disability may have to be detected by subjective evaluations rather than by objectively validated tests. In many cases the educator may provide a series of well-planned, systematically organized anecdotes about a child's daily behavior to evoke the fundamental information that will permit a useful evaluation to be made.

The emotional characteristics of gifted/learning disabled children cannot be considered unique. The differences between them and other learning disabled pupils seem to be in the intensity of their defenses. It is as if they were bringing their intelligence to bear on not solving the problem. They divert their energy from learning to maintaining the defenses.

Denial, projection, and rationalization are favored defense mechanisms since each tends to reduce guilt and fear. Parents often are caught up in the same defenses and in some cases, such as those involving rationalization, are apt to pass them on to their children.

Behaviorally, gifted/learning disabled children, unlike their achieving peers, tend to use passive-aggressive techniques. These can cause serious difficulties for teachers and parents since there is no real resistance to work against. Eventually a decision must be made about these behaviors: Are they amenable to educational alteration or are they so devastating to learning that only psychological intervention can save the situation?

REFERENCE

Abrams, J.A. A psychodynamic understanding of the emotional aspects of learning disorders. In *Advances in special education* (Vol. 2). Greenwich, Conn.: JAI Press, Inc., 1980, pp. 29-50.

SUGGESTED READINGS

Abrams, J.A. Parental dynamics—their role in learning disabilities. *The reading teacher,* 1970, *23,* 751-760.

Adamson, W. Individual psychotherapy. In *A handbook for specific learning disabilities.* New York: Gardner Press, 1978.

Blanchard, P. Psychoanalytic contribution to the problems of reading disability. *Psychoanalytic study of the child,* 1964, *2,* 163-187.

Harris, I. *Emotional blocks to learning.* New York: The Free Press, 1961.

Vogel, E.F., & Bell, N.W. The emotionally disturbed child as the family scapegoat. In *The family.* New York: The Free Press, 1968.

Chapter 3

Diagnostic Aspects

As noted earlier, a major problem in dealing with the gifted/learning disabled child is the concept that the usual diagnostic tests and procedures used with average pupils are valid. As of this writing, there appears to be no evidence that this is true. The effects of superior intelligence on testing outcomes appear to be underinvestigated.

PROBLEMS IN CURRENT PRACTICES

The problem is, of course, intensified by diagnostic practices and resulting recommendations based on standardized achievement tests. Two major factors cloud the issue but too frequently are unperceived or ignored.

The first factor is that nearly all reading achievement tests tend to be power tests. That is, the test supposedly becomes harder the farther into it the student progresses. In and of itself, the concept is valid and useful but it may be less so when put into test development. For example, if a perfect power test could be built and a perfect child took it, the following useful results would happen.

The perfect child would move through the perfect test with perfect accuracy until reaching the first question that the pupil could not answer. At that point, the teacher would know that the child must stop because no more items could be answered correctly (because each question after this would be harder). Ergo: a perfect test. The child has reached a point in the test where nothing more can be done. In everyday life when someone can do no more, it is said that the point of frustration has been reached. This is equally true for the pupil taking the power achievement test. If the child gives all there is to give on the test, the point of frustration must be reached. Interestingly, if this does not happen, the power test is of little value for evaluation.

However, there are no perfect tests, nor perfect children. A number of confounding things occur. Some children do know answers beyond their first failure. On multiple choice items children guess, unwisely and wildly (so, of course, do adults). In such situations, the score often represents a point beyond frustration yet is accepted as being diagnostically meaningful.

The second factor clouding the diagnostic issue is the test result itself. Nearly all achievement tests can produce a grade-level score. How frequently are these scores translated directly into reader level values? For years a common standard for determining reading retardation was a child's score on a reading achievement test two or more grade levels below grade level placement. The scientific proof of this contrast is unknown yet its acceptance has placed children into instructional programs in reading when their needs were in basic language skills. This simple relationship has had terrible consequences. On the other hand, this equating of achievement and grade level has been used to label as gifted some children who, in effect, may simply be better-than-average readers.

The pronounced danger in using this equation for the gifted/learning disabled is that it often fails to identify children operating at grade level who have a real potential for greater achievement. Since they are performing "satisfactorily," little is done to help them achieve their true potential.

DETERMINING POTENTIAL AND ACHIEVEMENT

Informal Reading Inventory

If the gifted/learning disabled child is to be recognized and have appropriate needs met, it is important to look at behaviors in actual practice rather than on tests. Informal appraisals offer far more information that can be used than do standardized measures. Too frequently, an IQ score of 130 or higher is interpreted to mean that a child has superior potential in all areas of existence and all facets of education. Educators who have worked with very bright children know that the youngsters are not uniformly gifted. They may demonstrate above-average ability across the academic spectrum but the giftedness tends to be rather specific. Therefore, it is vital to measure whether or not reading retardation does exist.

An informal reading inventory technique is most helpful (Johnson & Kress, 1965). It is important to determine at what level a child could be expected to read and compare it with the one where there would be profit from instruction. Therefore, in using an informal reading inventory, educators need to ascertain the instructional level in the material used and compare it with the listening comprehension level. The basic assumption is that if children can understand, with 75 percent comprehension, a piece of material read to them aloud, they should be able to read and understand it by themselves. Reading retardation is simply the difference between listening comprehension and reading comprehension (Betts, 1946).

This fundamental procedure, of course, eliminates the confounding factors of intelligence, grade level, past experience, etc., and provides the examiner with clear-cut data. Through its use, the teacher can be made aware of the fact that retardation in one type of reading may differ markedly from retardation in another. This recognition is especially important for very bright children, because they often have areas of intense interest in which they can demonstrate outstanding performances. This evaluation concept deserves further credence since it requires all who deal with the child to recognize that reading is a processing of something, not something in and of itself. The value of this information in planning an instructional program cannot be minimized.

A detailed subjective analysis of performance on the informal reading inventory can provide insight into skills or problems in attitude toward reading, word attack skills (Chapter 7), general comprehension abilities, and organizational skills. Since the inventory may use literature, social science, physical science, or functional materials, educators can discover abilities or inabilities appropriate to these areas. This information provides an understanding of strengths that can be drawn upon and problems that need solving.

Tests of Memory Span

An important element in being successful in academic tasks is the ability to deal with data presented sequentially. It also is necessary to be able to retain a series of knowns to use as resources when trying to deal with unknowns. Individuals frequently need to move in an organized, systematic manner to solve a problem. All of these procedures require memory or delayed recall. However, before memory comes memory span. How much information can a person confront at a presentation before becoming unable to encompass any more or having to give up on data presented previously? This is the realm of memory span or immediate recall. How long can a sentence be before a person forgets the beginning or cannot tolerate any more words? How many unrelated words can be said before the hearer cannot repeat them? (When a President of the United States is sworn in, the Chief Justice reads the oath in groups of only four to six words.) What is the memory span for digits forward or digits reversed?

Memory span and its effects often are neglected for all children. The gifted/learning disabled may never have their abilities in this area appraised either directly or informally. In far too many cases a valid intelligence test is administered but only the total score is reported to the teaching staff. Pronounced problems in digit span or arithmetic might be evident in the subtest scaled scores but these scores are not revealed. The child then may be placed in a program in which the demands on memory span preclude success. However, the same program, with a deliberate modification of the amount of material presented at one time in an area and in a combination of areas, might well have been successful. A child who is superior in a global sense may still have a handicap in trying to deal with extended series of words, sentences, or ideas.

The *Detroit Tests of Learning Aptitude* (Baker & Leland, 1967) offer on a standardized basis a number of useful analyses. Test 6, "Auditory Attention Span for Unrelated Words," and test 9, "Visual Attention Span for Objects," both deal with discrete, unorganized data presented aurally and visually. Both tests supply a weighted score that, when compared to the simple mental age score, provides an interesting measure of the pupil's persistence when involved with a frustrating task. It may well be that some of the lack of adaptability in some gifted/learning disabled children noted earlier is a product of this inability to persist.

Test 13, "Auditory Attention Span for Related Syllables," presents sentences of increasing length. The student must repeat them as accurately as possible to the examiner. Three errors in a sentence are considered a failure. The results again can be computed to give a mental age. An internal analysis of the data will show the examiner just how much data can be presented in a meaningful sequence to a child before memory span proves inadequate.

How often are bright children chided for not following oral directions or completing assigned tasks? Parents often repeat the same charges about behavior at home. In nearly all cases, the child's brightness is emphasized but the ability to deal with a piece of extended conversation is unevaluated. Some of the maladjustment of the gifted/learning disabled might stem, understandably, from their inability to deal with lengthy sequential material in a manner commensurate with overall intelligence.

Test 18, "Oral Directions," follows the same basic procedure but the sentences are steps in a direction for which a motor production is required after all the directions are given. Without investigating in detail, is it possible to know whether an inadequate performance is attributable to poor attitude or a basic disability in holding a number of directions in mind and then using them appropriately? Too frequently the child's brightness causes investigators to overlook these relevant facts.

Informal Evaluations of Classification Skills

Many of the gifted/learning disabled, as noted earlier, are poor in adaptability and versatility. One of the best ways to evaluate the child in these areas is with informal measures of classification abilities. (See Chapter 8.)

The first skill to be measured is the ability to abstract. A simple verbal problem is presented to the child:

"Without looking, what are the parts of a chair?"

If there is difficulty in responding, the child should be allowed to look at a chair and name its parts. The teacher presents other objects to discover whether the child can tell the functions, parts, color, etc. A number of bright children find this difficult. An overall appraisal also is available in the Similarities Subtest of the Wechsler Intelligence Tests (Wechsler, 1974). If that subtest is used, the teacher should conduct a subjective analysis for the internal scatter. (Internal scatter is an inconsistent pattern of correct and incorrect responses.) Many gifted/learning disabled children will show such a result.

Another important measure is obtained from the following task:

Teacher: Look at these words and put them into two groups.

bus	car	canoe
raccoon	bear	dog
cat	raft	

The teacher should note the child's procedure in performing the task. Once it is completed, the teacher should ask the child how the groupings were made. At this time there is no need to call for a classification. If the child is unsuccessful, an instructional program should be set up to meet this very crucial need. If the child has been successful, the teacher should use the same words but require that they be put into four groups. (See Chapter 8 on developing classification skills.)

For many gifted/learning disabled children this demand to be adaptable and versatile is noticeably frustrating. In effect, two groups emerge: (1) those unable to classify and (2) those unable to be versatile in their classification.

These findings have much impact for instructional planning and prognosis. In some cases the inability to handle classification tasks may be the major cause of limited success in school.

The classification task that logically would follow these evaluation techniques provides insight into type and depth of vocabulary and versatility in its application—a vocabulary problem noted earlier.

Intelligence Tests

It is not necessary to become an expert administrator of the widely accepted *Wechsler Intelligence Scale for Children* (Wechsler, 1974) as a measure of potential to use its results. In a study of more than 450 children with reading problems and an intelligence quotient higher than 125, some interesting data emerged (Fox, 1981). While a detailed analysis still was being conducted at this writing, some of the initial findings corroborated insights from the author's personal experience with gifted/learning disabled children:

- A total score on the verbal, performance, or full-scale classification may not be as helpful as the scaled score results of certain subtests.
- The verbal score in academic areas tends to indicate children who should be making better progress than the performance score.
- The score on the similarities subtest for the gifted/learning disabled often is the highest. This test seems to pinpoint their better-than-average ability to form concepts.
- The score on the information subtest, while possibly better than average, often is four to six points lower than similarities.
- The vocabulary subtest score usually is a little higher than information but again noticeably lower than similarities.
- The two measures of attention and concentration, the digits and arithmetic subtests, tend to produce the lowest scores.

There is some basic pragmatic realism that might account for these performances. In many cases, the similarities subtest does represent the ability to form concepts, a characteristic that can be indicative of intelligence, while both the information and vocabulary subtests depend to a large degree on the cultural wealth of early schooling experience (Rapaport, Gill, & Schafer, 1968).

Children with learning disabilities usually lack such wealth in their early schooling. The emphasis on skills to the neglect of content that is typical of remedial programs would seem to make the differences in the performances on these tests self-evident. Performance on the digit span and arithmetic subtests is strongly affected by anxiety. Most gifted/learning disabled children tend to demonstrate anxiety as a result of the polarizing of their situation: overall ability vs. specific lack of achievement. The school and home pressures on these children because of their lack of success are debilitating, and are usually reflected in their performance. A valuable source of insight is the Rapaport, Gill, and Schafer book noted above.

At this point it is necessary to turn to speculation. Gifted/underachievers might not demonstrate the patterns just noted. Some educators feel that pattern analysis has no place in categorizing children. However, on a purely subjective basis, it seems apparent that gifted/learning disabled pupils would be placed in sociological and psychological circumstances that would readily foster those subtest patterns while the gifted/underachievers would not, simply because the type and amount of external pressure would be more limited and the internal pressure from self-doubt could be rationalized easily. The disabled child cannot do; the under-achiever does not do. The factor of volition cannot be ignored.

DIAGNOSTIC OBSERVATION AND TEACHING

Before any decisions are made about labeling and placement of children who might be considered handicapped, the subjective perceptions of skilled teachers must be considered. Too frequently, decisions are made using numbers or patterns alone. Such total objectivity often lacks many vital elements that are necessary for providing the most effective services.

One aspect of assessment usually overlooked is diagnostic observation. The learning disabilities teacher should observe the behavior of a child in a particular instructional situation and related social contacts. Attitudes, interests, and specific behavior in terms of skills, vocabulary, and concepts should be noted as well as teacher-child, child-to-child, and child-to-group interactions. Once giftedness appears to be a factor, each teacher's individual observations about the behaviors and interactions should be compared and contrasted. From these joint observa-tions, a short-term instructional program should be developed.

Using the short-term plan as the format, the learning disabilities instructor should initiate a series of diagnostic teaching activities, with appropriate contribu-tions from the gifted specialist. It is important in diagnostic teaching to present something different. A simple redoing of things already done is of no value. New ways of presenting materials, new materials, different groupings, and multisen-sory approaches should be tried. This should not imply a radical change in the program. Good programming would have these by definition; they would be new only to the child being evaluated.

To accomplish these tasks and obtain the best results, teachers must be objec-tively subjective—using subjective observations as objectively as possible. If the problem is based on an unsatisfactory pupil-teacher or group interaction, some professional must understand this and make the appropriate adjustments. If the matter is simply faulty assessment or programming, that fact must be communi-cated to those capable of making change. If the problem is real, if there is a real disability, then direct programmatic changes must be suggested by the assigned observer, and those responsible for such alterations should begin making them.

In most cases the agent of change is the school principal. If the child is both gifted and learning disabled, the task can become formidable. (See Chapter 17 on administrators' responsibilities.) However, the difficulties in developing a pro-gram for gifted/learning disabled children do not excuse administrators from the responsibility to provide one.

SUMMARY

To do total justice to the diagnosis of the gifted/learning disabled would require an entire book. Although most teachers do not have the training or professional inclination to be professional diagnosticians, they can learn to interpret test results and make use of the information in planning a program.

An informal measure of reading ability or an informal reading inventory can measure the differences between aural language ability and reading ability. This can be used as a measure of retardation in reading. This difference will vary in different curricula and interest areas.

The memory span ability can be determined since this element permeates so many other academic and psychological processes. The different aspects of this one ability must be delineated.

Informal measures of classification ability can be employed. This area often is neglected yet it is a major element in concept formation that is a big problem for many learning disabled children.

With some training, teachers can appraise these three areas. However, most teachers are not trained to administer or interpret the Wechsler Intelligence Scale for Children. With further training, teachers can appreciate the meaning of the performances on certain subscales, their scaled scores, and the interaction implied by combinations of scores.

Finally, the very important roles of diagnostic observation and teaching must be developed in teachers. An orderly process involving both components is vital for best placement and programming. However, the problems of poor ego and low self-esteem generated in the adult world by these diagnostic aspects of the gifted/learning disabled program cannot be minimized.

REFERENCES

Baker, H., & Leland, B. *Detroit tests of learning aptitude*. Indianapolis: The Bobbs-Merrill Company, Inc., 1967.

Betts, C.A. *Foundations of reading instruction*. New York: American Book Company, 1946.

Fox, Lynn. Gifted children with learning disabilities: An analysis. Paper presented at the Colloquium on gifted/learning disabled children, The Johns Hopkins University, Baltimore, 1981.

Johnson, M.S., & Kress, R.A. *Informal reading inventories*. Newark, Del.: International Reading Association, 1965.

Rapaport, D., Gill, M., & Schafer, R. *Diagnostic psychological testing*. New York International University Press, Inc., 1968.

Wechsler, D. *Manual for the Wechsler intelligence scale for children, revised*. New York: The Psychological Corporation, 1974.

SUGGESTED READINGS

Anderson, M., Kaufman, A., & Kaufman, N. Use of the WISC-R with a learning disabled population: Some diagnostic implications. *Psychology in the Schools,* 1976, *13*(4).

Bannatyne, A. Diagnosing learning disabilities and writing remedial prescriptions. *Journal of Learning Disabilities,* 1968, *1*(4).

Elkind, J. The gifted child with learning disabilities. *The Gifted Child Quarterly,* 1973, *17*(2).

Frierson, E. The gifted child with special learning disabilities. *Learning Disorders,* 1968, *3*.

Gallagher, J.J. Issues in education for the gifted. In H. Passow (Ed.), *The gifted and the talented: Their education development,* 78th yearbook of the National Society for the Study of Education. Chicago: University of Chicago Press, 1979.

Karnes, M., McCoy, G., Zehrbach, R., Wollersheim, J., & Clarizio, H. The efficacy of two organizational plans for underachieving intellectually gifted children. *Exceptional Children,* 1963.

Kaufman, A.S. A new approach to the interpretation of test scatter on the WISC-R. *Journal of Learning Disabilities,* 1976, *9*(3).

Maker, C.J. *Providing programs for the gifted handicapped.* Reston, Va.: The Council for Exceptional Children, 1977.

Meisgeier, C., Meisgeier, C., & Werblo, D. Factors compounding the handicapping of some children. *The Gifted Child Quarterly,* 1978, *22*(3).

Vance, H., Gaynor, P., & Coleman, M. Analysis of cognitive abilities for learning disabled children. *Psychology in the Schools,* 1976, *13*(4).

Vance, H., & Singer, M. Recategorization of the WISC-R subtest scaled scores for learning disabled children. *Journal of Learning Disabilities,* 1979, *12*(8).

Whitmore, J. *Giftedness, conflict, and underachievement.* Boston: Allyn & Bacon, Inc., 1980.

Chapter 4

Early Identification

Early identification of all cognitive exceptionalities has always been much more difficult than the detection of physical difficulties. Yet there have been increasing demands for early identification of giftedness and learning disabilities throughout the country and in many other parts of the world. Unfortunately, these demands often border on the simplistic.

Professionals have had problems in these areas for a couple of reasons. First, there really is not enough fundamental information about child development to make the inferences in these areas more nearly approach fact. Second, the instruments used in many cases are inadequate and in some instances are invalid. Interestingly, even when such invalidities are demonstrated, there is a real reluctance among professionals to drop these instruments, possibly because there are fewer instruments to substitute and many states required statistical measures. The concept of construct validity in these tests seldom is challenged. It is assumed that if the test makers say they test something, then the tests must test it. This blind faith has led to many serious mistakes in diagnosis and programming for both gifted and learning disabled children.

IDENTIFICATION OF GIFTEDNESS

In the early identification of giftedness, a number of elements must be balanced. First, it appears that the opportunity to display giftedness is vital if that talent is to be perceived. Children in very sterile environments with no opportunity for challenge cannot rise to opportunities. This rise is a characteristic of gifted children. Second, most of the perceptions that alert others to the giftedness in children initially are observational. This means that the observer must know child development and look for examples of precocity. A short list of cognitive and language milestones follows this chapter. (See Appendix 4-A.)

27

Since the child spends these early years for the most part in the home, the parents' sensitivity is crucial. Parents must be provided with information and techniques for observing the child and recording anecdotes. The importance of good anecdotal recordkeeping for the early identification of giftedness cannot be overestimated.

The other key aspect of early identification involves formalized testing, an area in which great discretion is required. The problem with validity has been noted; there also is difficulty with reliability.

In many formalized programs for early identification of giftedness, standardized tests are used and judgments are based on normative scores. This approach often is not satisfactory for gifted children, for a number of reasons:

- Gifted children tend to be inquisitive even at an early age and may not stay with tasks long enough to demonstrate their true potential in any area being measured.
- These children tend to have specific interests and often will not go ahead with a task for which they see no reward. It must be remembered that they have not yet adopted the pleasure-pain principle.
- Tests often have such a low upper limit that gifted and nongifted children cannot be distinguished.

These problems are especially acute in reading readiness tests. Many gifted children are already reading before they enter school and many of the subtests appear to be superfluous to them. Unfortunately, their scores are interpreted as indicating lack of mastery, so skills programs are initiated. There is little recognition in the school community that successful reading is a demonstration of skills mastery. Bright children usually develop their own cognitive approaches to reading tasks and often they do not conform to a school's skill sequences. Many of these children have been seriously damaged because of this lack of recognition.

If standardized measures are to be used, it is important to look at the internal performances on these tests. What these children did usually is more valuable for analysis than what they did not do. Several indicators of precocity should alert adults in the children's lives to develop a more formal approach to the identification of possible giftedness including intelligence and creativity testing. The internal subjective analysis of standardized tests is a fundamental prerequisite to early identification.

This statement can cause a problem in many schools. If the early identification process, or even the reading readiness evaluation, is carried out with tests that are scored by machine and recorded by computers, then subjective evaluations cannot be made. Every school system needs tests that are not used systemwide. If giftedness is suspected, some staff member should be empowered to administer, score, and evaluate an individual test of whatever nature is needed. These results plus any anecdotal reports developed by the teacher during the testing should receive the most credence in moving toward the identification of giftedness. This entire strategy implies that this type of evaluation can only occur individually or in groups of less than four. The teacher must observe the performances and note significant behaviors and comments during the test.

The person responsible for evaluating the children must be able to choose achievement-appropriate, not grade-appropriate, measures. In this way tests can be used with enough upper limits to ensure that decision making is more accurate. There is, of course, a danger in this approach since what eventually is tested is the depth of the children's background of experience. Since they have not lived very long, that background, although not meager, is limited. It is because of this element that the teacher's anecdotal notes concerning the type and depth of thinking must be correlated with all test results.

It usually is helpful to use a more formalized test of intelligence to obtain a satisfactory evaluation. For young children, the Wechsler Preschool and Primary Scale of Intelligence (WPPSI) (Wechsler, 1967) is highly recommended since it provides a full testing scale as well as verbal and performance intelligence quotients. Since subtest scaled scores are provided, it also provides an opportunity for teachers to perceive both particularly strong aspects and relatively weak or poor elements of intellectual function. This is important since a full-scale score might indicate giftedness yet an analysis of the subtests may reveal that most of the score is influenced by a high performance rating.

This type of child might lead a miserable life in many gifted programs in which the emphasis is on verbal facility. In a program designed to use those elements of the performance type of giftedness, the child could become highly motivated and productive. Patterns of subtests and their significance have been analyzed by a number of researchers and are worthy of note (Anderson, A. Kaufman, & N. Kaufman, 1976; A.S. Kaufman, 1976; Vance & Singer, 1979).

IDENTIFICATION OF LEARNING DISABILITIES

Early identification of learning disabilities poses a different set of problems. One of the most difficult is that of disability vs. inability. The opportunity to rise to challenges is not as important in this case as is the opportunity for any challenges at all. If no opportunity is presented, it cannot be determined whether the child could or could not face it. Therefore, in the evaluation of possible learning disability early in life, the family and community background must be understood. (See Chapter 5.)

The difficulty is further compounded by the law that states that learning disability cannot be diagnosed in cases where the condition is the result of social, economic, or cultural deprivation (P.L. 94-142). It is easier, programmatically and financially, for schools to ascribe poor early test results to those factors rather than investigating the possibility of a disability.

Once again, the early identification of learning disability is best carried out in the home. The developmental milestones at the end of this chapter can be helpful but too often this type of information is not available to most people.

Parents must be helped. This often is best done as a community effort to assist them in becoming better observers of behavior and keepers of records. However, in many homes, circumstances may well make such procedures impossible.

Because of these problems, nursery school and kindergarten teachers must be particularly alert to factors involved with learning disabilities. Some of these involve children's:

- inability to adjust to new situations or tasks
- lack of interest in verbal activities or numbers
- difficulty in dealing with time factors
- inability to see beyond the whole to the parts
- failure to demonstrate language growth and vocabulary acquisition
- lack of versatility in appropriate responses to varying situations

IDENTIFICATION OF OPPORTUNITIES

Another early identification problem deals with opportunity. There is good evidence that maturation is required, especially in the central nervous system, before certain types of tasks can be learned. This is true of many cognitive processes such as reading, writing, and numerical manipulation. Consequently, it is inappropriate to ask these tasks of children below the age of four. Therefore, disabilities in these areas usually do not appear until the child is confronted with the tasks in school. Even in school, the problem of lack of maturation or of disability cannot be addressed easily simply because in most instances educators have neither the instruments nor the procedures to make a definitive decision. This, of course, means that delays in needed remediation or habilitation are common. These delays are not the result of professionals' indifference but are caused by their genuine concern about applying incorrect labels and procedures.

Therefore, it is vitally important that kindergarten programs introduce some reading and arithmetic instruction on a diagnostic/prescriptive basis. If observable problems are noted, especially for children who have passed through the developmental milestones rather well, special attention should be paid to these pupils as possible candidates for preventive programs. Of course, those who have not passed the developmental milestones consistently should be provided with as much diagnostic help as possible and remediation should be automatic.

IDENTIFICATION OF COGNITIVE PROBLEMS

The early identification of difficulties with cognitive processing is truly a problem within a dilemma. In many instances false positive identification can be as destructive as false negative identification. Yet either identification can be justified at times on the basis of observation and data and still reflect honest effort.

Parent and teacher information, observation, and detailed notation are the best means available for early identification. Formalized testing and diagnosis never can replace those three components. That is why most early identification programs that are totally based on school testing are automatically too late.

Early identification of gifted/learning disabled children is even more difficult than identifying one exceptionality alone. Precocity in passing milestones can be demonstrated by children who then are subjected to academic tasks for which they may not be maturationally ready. Emotional problems are developed because of this, and school failure follows. Maturation may even have occurred but the adjustment difficulties preclude learning. The child is labeled learning disabled although in truth the learning problem stems from emotionality. This one element in evaluating gifted children who are not succeeding cannot be overlooked.

For children who have demonstrated possible giftedness at an early age, special attention should be given to the six factors listed earlier for recognizing learning disability. If these elements are obvious in the child's behavior, there is reason for concern. This concern should be expressed in obtaining more detailed physical, psychological, and intellectual evaluations. All three areas must be investigated and a good multidisciplinary diagnosis obtained. Such evaluations can be obtained at teaching hospitals and clinics. If only one aspect of the child's life is examined, little help probably will be forthcoming.

Precocity in one area may not reflect overall giftedness. Some authorities feel it should be interpreted that way. However, this interpretation often leads to unhappiness and discontent for both children and family. Too frequently gifted readers are not precocious in other areas and yet have unreasonable demands made on them by others. In another instance, children with particular abilities are labeled handicapped because they do not reach the same level of achievement in all areas. These rather normal children then are subjected to programs designed for problem pupils that in no way address their needs. In some cases children have had a complete loss of self-esteem because of programs seeking to force them to deal with nonexistent problems. The early identification of giftedness may be very destructive to pupils if the parents and school do not maintain the perspective that they are dealing with a developing organism with many areas—a child. When the parents' needs supersede the child's, suffering usually is the outcome.

SUMMARY

Early identification of giftedness or learning disabilities is not easy or exact. The psychosocial interactions of young children offer so many alternatives and possibilities that precise perceptions are nearly impossible.

Systematic, knowledgeable observations are vital. These must be followed by systematic multidisciplinary evaluation procedures that will generate a number of possible remedial or habilitative procedures. The opportunities for attempting the suggested procedures must be available and free of pressure. (See Chapter 14 on the teacher as learning therapist.)

Finally, the parents, who will be the most help in early identification, need information and guidance and must be accepted by the professionals as being reasonable as well as concerned. Parents must understand that the state of the art in early identification prevents the professionals from being totally decisive. They are not talking out of both sides of their mouths but are describing possible alternative interpretations of findings. Parents also must attempt to achieve as much objectivity as possible about their child. They should not use the child as the fulfillment of their ego needs. They must accept the child.

If exceptionalities are suspected, professional help always should be sought as early as possible. Truth is better than fiction or fantasy in helping a child become a happy, adjusted, productive human being.

REFERENCES

Anderson, M., Kaufman, A., & Kaufman, N. Use of the WISC-R with a learning disabled population: Some diagnostic implications. *Psychology in the Schools,* 1976, *13*(4), 381-386.

Kaufman, A.S. A new approach to the interpretation of test scatter on the WISC-R. *Journal of Learning Disabilities,* 1976, *9*(3), 160-168.

Public Law 94-142, the *Education for All Handicapped Children Act of 1975,* Sec. 620(b)(4)(A), 89 Stat. 794.

Vance, H., & Singer, M. Recategorization of the WISC-R subtest scaled scores for learning disabled children. *Journal of Learning Disabilities,* 1979, *12*(8), 487-491.

Vulpe, S.G. *Vulpe assessment battery.* Toronto: National Institute on Mental Retardation, 1977.

Wechsler, D. *Manual for the Wechsler preschool and primary scale of intelligence.* New York: The Psychological Corporation, 1967.

SUGGESTED READINGS

Adelman, H.S. Predicting psychoeducational problems in childhood. *Behavioral Disorders,* 1978, *3*(3), 148-159.

Becker, L.D., & Snider, M.A. Teachers' ratings and predicting special class placement. *Journal of Learning Disabilities,* 1979, *12*(2), 96-99.

Beers, C.S., & Beers, J.W. Early identification of learning disabilities: Facts and fallacies. *Elementary School Journal,* 1980, *81*(2), 67-76.

Behar, L.B. The preschool behavior questionnaire. *Journal of Abnormal Child Psychology,* 1977, *5*(3), 265-275.

Buch, C.B. Recent insights on the culturally different gifted. *The Gifted Child Quarterly,* 1978, *22*(3), 374-392.

Colarusso, R.P. Teacher effectiveness in identifying high-risk kindergarten children. *Journal of Learning Disabilities,* 1979, *12*(10), 684-86.

Coles, G.S. The learning disabilities test battery: Empirical and social issues. *Harvard Educational Review,* 1978, *48*(3), 313-340.

Cowgill, N.L., Friedland, S., & Shapiro, R. Predicting learning disabilities from kindergarten reports. *Journal of Learning Disabilities,* 1973, *6,* 577-582.

Crow, G.A. *Children at risk: A handbook of the signs and symptoms of early childhood difficulties.* New York: Shocken Books, 1978.

Ferinden, W.E., & Jacobson, S. Early identification of learning disabilities. *Journal of Learning Disabilities,* 1979, *3*(11), 589-593.

Hall, E. Knowing who is gifted. *Gifted Child Journal,* 1980, *2*(11), 14-15, 50-51.

Hoffman, M.S. Early identification of learning problems. *Academic Therapy Quarterly,* 1971, *7,* 23-35.

Karnes, M.B., & Bertscki, J.D. Identifying and educating gifted/talented nonhandicapped and handicapped preschoolers. *Teaching Exceptional Children,* 1978, *10*(4), 114-119.

Keogh, B. Early identification of children with potential learning problems. *The Journal of Special Education,* 1970, *4,* 349-356.

Keogh, B.K., & Becker, L. Early detection of learning problems: Questions, cautions, and guidelines. *Exceptional Children,* 1973, *40,* 5-11.

Kochanek, T.T. Early detection programs for preschool handicapped children: Some procedural recommendations. *The Journal of Special Education,* 1980, *14*(3), 347-353.

Landig, H.J., & Naumann, T.F. Aspects of intelligence in gifted preschoolers. *The Gifted Child Quarterly,* 1978, *22*(1), 85-89.

Lansdown, R. The learning disabled child: Early detection and prevention. *Developmental Medicine and Child Neurology,* 1978, *20*(4), 496-497.

Lewis, A. The early identification of children with learning difficulties. *Journal of Learning Disabilities,* 1980, *13*(2), 102-108.

Mercer, C.D. Early identification: Issues and considerations. *Exceptional Children,* 1979, *46*(1), 52-55.

Mercer, C.D., & Trifiletti, J.J. The development of screening procedures for the early detection of children with learning problems. *Journal of School Health,* 1977, *47*(9), 526-532.

Satz, P., & Fletcher, J. Early screening tests: Some uses and abuses. *Journal of Learning Disabilities,* 1978, *11*(6), 347-351.

Shorr, D.N., Jackson, N.E., & Robinson, H.B. Achievement test performance of intellectually advanced preschool children. *Exceptional Children,* 1979, *17*(3), 18-19.

Appendix 4-A

Developmental Scale in Language and Related Factors

To provide a detailed developmental scale in language and related areas would require an entire book, and, in fact, it has been done: a very detailed assessment battery is published by the Canadian National Institute on Mental Retardation as the *Vulpe Assessment Battery* (Vulpe, 1977). It is so detailed, however, that it probably is more useful for professionals than parents.

The condensed version presented here is not intended to be as definitive. It is hoped that the categories are broad enough and yet contain enough detail that parents can use it to alert themselves to possible problems or precocities. The detailed analysis and diagnosis should be carried out by appropriately trained professionals. The scale proposes that the child:

Through 12 months:

- uses three to five words with correct meaning—family names, foods, etc.
- makes many different sounds; seems to enjoy random vocalization
- "talks" to toys, stuffed animals, etc.

Through 24 months:

- uses language on a greater scale
- indicates desires and requirements
- names concrete objects and items in pictures
- has larger listening vocabulary than speaking vocabulary
- begins questioning for information
- uses two-word or three-word sentences, especially for requests
- increases speaking vocabulary (Authorities disagree on number—40 as a minimum or as high as 750—but do agree that most words used are nouns, with some prepositions.)

- answers questions correctly
- uses a few personal pronouns correctly
- enjoys looking at books and being read to

Through 36 months:

- begins to name colors
- provides full name
- uses nearly all the appropriate vowels and many of the consonants
- improves overall articulation
- sings songs and enjoys doing it
- tells and retells stories
- recalls happenings from the recent past
- begins to use "you" correctly
- expands spoken vocabulary to between 500 and 1,000 words (The experts again disagree on number.)
- looks at books alone for pleasure
- knows some nursery rhymes
- begins to count by rote
- names most body parts
- recognizes own sex

Through 48 months:

- uses complete sentences but still may falter on grammatical correctness
- speaks fluently
- identifies the use of objects such as utensils, tools, etc.
- masters plurals
- uses sentences of longer duration—seven, eight, nine words in length
- speaks of future—"tomorrow," "when I get older," etc.
- participates in conversations
- knows names of most colors
- uses negatives very strongly
- scribbles with crayons
- likes to draw and produces recognizable work
- reverses letters when copying
- begins to establish directionality of left and right

- asks many "why" and "how" questions
- begins to recognize fact from fantasy
- begins to cooperate in group play or activities

Through 60 months:

- repeats days of week correctly
- describes objects with a number of attributes
- asks meanings of words
- knows home address and telephone number
- knows birthdate
- listens to and retells long stories
- counts by rote beyond ten
- writes numbers through ten
- demonstrates independent learning of words
- uses all parts of speech, including irregularities
- converses for extended periods of time
- understands parts of objects, such as half, etc.
- recognizes some coins
- knows morning, evening, day, night, etc.

Chapter 5

The Socioeconomically Deprived Child

When attempts are made at categorizing human beings, the results always must be questioned. So many uniquely human factors must be excluded that all of these generalizations become doubtful. Giftedness and learning disabilities suffer the same fate.

Do intelligence tests measure intelligence? Do achievement tests measure achievement for children with problems? What is talent? Is it not in the eye of the beholder? Does lack of language ability limit the potential of a child? Can it be overcome?

All of these dilemmas—and they truly are dilemmas—surface with one important segment of the population: the socioeconomically disadvantaged. If it is assumed that traits are dispersed in a normal fashion across all populations, then the percentages for giftedness and learning disability also should be distributed normally. However, from pragmatic evidence, that does not appear to be true for giftedness if existing programs in schools are investigated. It is quite evident that the bulk of the gifted children must be verbally facile to be enrolled in gifted programs.

This does not appear to be a type of discrimination since with verbally facile children statistical documentation of giftedness can be obtained. For children who lack language facility, admission to gifted programs on subjective bases also would require that advantaged children who performed as well also be entered in a program that should have precise goals.

Socioeconomically deprived children can be eliminated from learning disabilities programs from a legal standpoint. In the definition of learning disabilities quoted in Chapter 1 (P.L. 94-142), it is apparent that a child must be excluded if the problem stems from environment, cultural, or economic disadvantage. However, since there really are no tests to indicate when these factors have or have not impinged on the child, it becomes legally safer to ascribe the problem to these elements rather than to confront the problem of proving the disability, once again with inadequate instruments. In times of diminishing funding, most services might well be provided to children by this route.

Although often in disrepute in today's totally legalistic approach to life, logic would seem to say that in the disadvantaged population there are gifted, learning disabled, and gifted/learning disabled children. The paradox is that a way must be found to delineate the first two before the third can be determined.

Regularly used evaluative and diagnostic procedures probably will color the examiner's view of the child. It is suggested here that a possible route for delineating disadvantaged children lies in a subjective/objective diagnostic observation and teaching approach. This concept, which admittedly is untried as a total approach, might be effective. Certain elements are absolutely necessary:

- The children in the program should have demonstrated in some documentable form thinking skills that have overridden experience and language barriers.
- A teacher trained in giftedness and learning disabilities should be assigned to work with this selected, selective group.
- The teacher, during the diagnostic activity, must be allowed to deviate from skill sequences and curriculum goals.
- The teacher's subjective evaluations must be accepted and the children put into appropriate programs. This acceptance, however, must at all times be stated as high-level, documented opinion and not be claimed to be fact. If this suggested program is to succeed, the teacher must not have to face threats of suit for malpractice or lack of due process or all of the other legalistic constraints on honest subjectivity.

To implement the program, the first approach should be one similar to that suggested in Chapter 11 on developing oral language facility. After the children have worked in it for a number of weeks, those who seem to have profited greatly should then begin to receive work in abstracting (described in detail in Chapter 8). Finally, the program in developing the use of context clues should be introduced. (See Chapter 7 on word recognition.)

As the selected group of children moves through these suggested programs, the teacher must be aware of those who seem to fall behind now that the more academic aspects are presented. The teacher should identify the child who has:

- trouble with time-related learning
- a tendency to use a limited, stilted vocabulary
- difficulty in recalling past events or retaining word learnings
- problems making adjustments in the program or seeing multiple approaches to tasks
- a need for much more time than others to complete a task

If these tendencies and other characteristics of learning disability are evident to the teacher, then the possibility of such a condition should be suggested. If the child has demonstrated ability to rise above the constraints of disadvantage in language functioning and then begins to falter seriously when academic procedures are introduced, the time for a more formal diagnostic program might have arrived. A more valid determination of giftedness should be available and specific tests for aspects of academic or learning disabilities should be used and evaluated.

The ultimate real value of this approach should be that the disadvantaged child is provided with a systematic opportunity to transcend the impediment. Educators and parents also would have a better understanding of the potential and needs of the child. Fact would replace illusion, probability could supplant hope, and realism could return to the child's life.

In all populations, another group of children always is mentioned as being undetected for specific help with giftedness: those with language-processing disorders. It seems evident that some pupils having this disorder must be gifted. However, as opposed to the socioeconomically disadvantaged, children with processing disorders are truly handicapped. Most of these problems are well beyond the range of skills, knowledge, and backgrounds of teachers—and rightly so. These children should, of course, be in a program designed by speech and language specialists to remediate or provide adaptation for the problem. Once these steps have been taken, it is useful for the children to work with a special educator. However, the only way the special educator can be of value initially is in the areas of diagnostic observation and diagnostic teaching.

It would be presumptuous in this text to suggest programs for children with disorders in language processing. That must be left to professionals who are trained to deal with this very puzzling and debilitating handicap. It is debatable whether gifted children with this disorder ever will really be able to use any gifted programs to reach their true potential.

SUGGESTED READINGS

Fantini, M.D. *The disadvantaged*. New York: Harper & Row, Publishers, 1968.

Hellmuth, J. *Disadvantaged child*. New York: Brunner/Mazel, Inc., 1967.

Public Law 94-142, the *Education for All Handicapped Children Act of 1975*, Sec. 620(b)(4)(A), 89 Stat. 794.

Riesman, F. *The culturally deprived child*. New York: Harper & Row, Publishers, 1962.

Williams, F. *Language and poverty*. Chicago: Markham Publishing Co., 1970.

Part II

Remediation Procedures Unit

Remediation procedures are presented in a general systematic format. It is assumed that readers are familiar with some of the techniques suggested but may not understand all of them. Therefore, the presentation advocates specific procedures in the appropriate places.

Chapter 6

Remediation Procedures

When developing a plan of action to meet the needs of gifted/learning disabled students, it is important to keep in the forefront of the effort the concept that prepackaged remedial programs are of little value. The strength of the program must rest on its individualization for the students. In the program suggested here, one concept must always be kept in mind: the need for independence of behavior. A major thesis of this plan is that all gifted and learning disabled children need to develop and to have independence. For them, independence should be the cornerstone of the program. The program exists to develop independence and needs it to thrive.

One of the most debilitating ideas about all children with problems is the one that keeps them dependent. A philosophy that requires them to have others do for them, of course, ultimately leads to a restricted, unsatisfying life style.

To deal with gifted/learning disabled children so as to allow them to reach their potential and make their contributions to society requires an effort to be supportive but not smothering.

THE FORMAT

If a child has a severe reading or writing problem, the following basic outline of procedures has been effective. The teacher:

- uses a modified language experience approach concerning a special interest of the child
- works out the ideas and language in an individual conference setting (see Appendix 6-A on integrative instruction)
- copies in good form the material to be developed by dictation from the student (see Appendix 6-A)

- directs the student to write the material and deal with errors using a multisensory word learning approach (see Appendix 6-C on a modified Fernald Procedure and Appendix 6-D on writing)
- prepares reinforcement and enrichment activities from the words generated by the writing (see Appendix 6-D)
- prepares the handwritten material in typed form for the student to read (see Appendix 6-D)
- notes errors anecdotally and deals with them as indicators for continued instruction (see Appendix 6-E on recordkeeping and anecdotal records)

Since each element or a combination of those listed is important, they are dealt with as separate entities. However, it must be noted that they cannot stand alone and are successful by reason of their integration as a totality.

A LANGUAGE EXPERIENCE APPROACH ✓

The language experience approach to reading and writing instruction has been a recognized instructional method for many years (Lamoreaux & Lee, 1943; Betts, 1946). Basically, the technique requires a child or children to dictate a story or article to the teacher, who in turn writes it down, usually on a large chart. This material is developed at the oral/aural stage before it is accepted for writing. However, it does not mean that in certain cases the teacher does not accept grammatical or syntactical imprecisions nor that jargon or slang does not appear. It usually represents the best oral performance the teacher can elicit at the time. Below is a sample of a language experience story written by a child with time sequencing problems:

I get up.
I put on my things.
I get washed.
I go down to eat.
I go to school.

This written material then becomes the vehicle for reading instruction. Since the concepts and vocabulary are the children's own, they minimize the difficulty commonly encountered in prepared material, and word attack and comprehension skills can be developed more easily. The goal, of course, is to use the language experience chart as the vehicle to move into prepared materials. However, it must be noted that it cannot be viewed as simply a beginning reading program. The concept is just as viable as a procedure for initiating successful reading at any level of sophistication. Those laboratory experiments in biology or chemistry that all educators had to perform and then write up were a modified language experience approach designed to enhance appreciation and understanding of a text or assigned reading. Too frequently, the technique is not viewed as sound preparation for any reading experience, but rather as an initial teaching activity.

The technique described often is called a total language experience approach since subject matter and vocabulary are taken basically intact from the students. However, it is possible to use the same fundamental procedure but modify it by using teacher goals in concepts and vocabulary. When this modification is employed, the technique is labeled a modified language experience approach. It is this latter procedure that seems best suited to the needs of the gifted/learning disabled student.

A MODIFIED LANGUAGE EXPERIENCE APPROACH

Since many such children have areas of intense interest or high sophistication, it is useful for the teacher to initiate the language experience approach with these areas. One important value is psychological. The learner may have had this interest thwarted for years because it did not fit into an appropriate place in the curriculum or it may have been too exotic for teachers to use in whole-class activities. The opportunity to pursue such an interest can counteract much of the negativism that often is characteristic of bright but frustrated children. The use of these ideas also can increase the chance for success and immediate recognition in reading and writing. Success and progress are absolutely vital to the long-term development of gifted/learning disabled children. The continuing failure they have suffered must be dealt with through short-term attainable goals. The best method for this is the use of a modified language experience approach based on a child's special interest.

Later, when success has become a rather regular occurrence, the move toward broadening interests will have to be made. Initially, the teacher must take advantage of the best hope of immediate success by accepting the idiosyncratic or exotic interests of the child. Failure to use this advantage probably will doom the remediation effort.

DEVELOPMENT OF THE CHARTS

The language experience chart for either type of approach should be designed to meet the needs of the readers. The fundamental difficulty concerns the status of the children who are going to use it. In one situation in which the children are illiterate or nearly so, or beginning or retarded readers, the language experience approach should be used to develop the ground rules for reading English. The following concepts must be integrated into the nervous system if reading as a process is to be understood:

1. that printed words in English represent sounds and that sounds represent meaning or reality
2. that words in writing are separated
3. that words and sentences are read from left to right in a line
4. that at the end of a line there is right-to-left and downward regression
5. that punctuation of a sentence is required

Each of these points needs some clarification. In Point 1, children must learn that words are symbols, not signs. Signs require no verbal mediation; symbols do. This implies that once the conversion of print to noise is made, the reader must convert the noise to a word. The reader or listener must do this. (See Chapter 7 on word recognition.)

For Point 2, it is important to note that in speech, spacing occurs by syllables, and a child should not be expected to recognize the differences between spoken and written word division. It also should be recalled that in earlier times English writing lacked spacing.

Point 3 represents a crucial understanding. When given a sequence of letters, pictures, etc., the normal procedure, if a person does not know the total sequence, is to move from one end to the other end, then to the middle. This is observed in many young children. Left-to-right progression, as in reading, really is an abnormality. It is a procedure determined, sociologically, not psychologically. Too frequently, this fact is not considered when reading instruction is initiated. The children must have this procedure embedded in their nervous systems, especially the eye muscles. For those who call left-to-right progression normal, it should be noted that children in Israel and the Arab world who are learning a Semitic language must learn to read right to left. Both groups of children, if they are to succeed in reading, must function with the appropriate abnormal process.

Point 4 again illustrates a sociological convention. There is really nothing organically correct about finishing a line of print and then moving to the next line by going right to left and downward. Watching children write is most helpful. When nonreaders begin writing words, they often go up or down the side of the paper when they reach the end of the line. (This is called the plowing method.) Others turn the page over. For many, the plowing method makes obvious sense. However, they must have right-to-left and downward regression firmly in their nervous systems.

Point 5 involves an obvious factor in written language processes. Punctuation is not used or needed in oral language (except as expressed in vocal pauses or emphases) but is required in writing to delineate sentences, suggest emphasis, indicate importance, etc. The major problem is that reading and writing involve two different psychological processes: (1) recognition of punctuation in reading and (2) its recall in writing. They can be difficult for any learning disabled child.

The Language Chart

Instruction with the language experience approach for beginning or severely retarded readers should be initiated with a language chart. This chart should be the vehicle for developing the know-how of reading English—the five points just discussed.

To provide the children with experience and develop their vocabulary, the teacher should have them dictate the material, then enter the dictated sentence on lined chart paper with black crayon in large manuscript writing.

While writing on the chart, the teacher should follow a basic procedure by vocalizing what is being done and why:

- "This is the title so all the words start with capital letters."
- "I must leave a space between each word."
- "This is the first sentence so I have to indent it, move it in."
- "The first word in the sentence always starts with a capital letter."
- "This is the end of the sentence. I must put a period—this dot—to show that the sentence is over."

It is important to encourage inductive learning throughout this procedure. Children who cannot yet read can be asked to show where one word ends or another begins or where a sentence starts or finishes. At all times the teacher must continue to return to the process of pronouncing the word and demonstrating that it must mean something.

Once a language chart is developed, one of the most important procedures must be initiated: left-to-right progression and right-to-left and downward regression. The teacher should discuss the ideas and vocabulary in the chart orally and aurally in a procedure such as this:

- Set up a purpose for the children's listening to the reading: "Listen to what I read and see if it is what we wanted to say yesterday."
- Begin reading the chart with a pointer.
- Draw the children's eyes across the page by moving the pointer in a smooth, continuous line while reading; there should not be a stop under each word.
- Reach the end of the line, then draw the children's eyes right to left on a diagonal to the beginning of the next line; however, in this move the teacher

should not say anything or provide any meaning (too often, a teacher begins saying the words on the next line before reaching there with the pointer).
- Follow this procedure until the chart is completed, then ask the children if there are any particular words or sentences they would like read; ask comprehension questions and reread correct answers to the group, but always with the smooth movement.

In this procedure, the children's eye muscles must acquire the concept that when the eyes move left to right there is meaning and sound but when they move right to left and downward there is no meaning or sound. Many teachers find it difficult to discipline themselves to avoid reading ahead of the pointer but it is absolutely necessary.

It would be interesting to note the number of learning disabled children demonstrating so-called reversal tendencies who never have learned how to follow the conventions of the English language. It should be remembered these procedures are arbitrary, not God-given.

After one or two rereadings following the suggested smooth-flow procedure, a new element can be introduced. The teacher can reread the material, putting the pointer under the middle of each word as it is pronounced. In the transition to the next line, the smooth flow with no sound or meaning is maintained.

The word-by-word procedure is the beginning of visual-auditory instruction for word learning. The children receive visual and auditory stimulation. After some instructional repetition, some of them, when asked, will begin to recognize words on demand, "Can you show me ___," and independently, "What word is that?" or "What word means big?"

At the point when some children begin to recognize words on their own, the language chart becomes a reading chart. The teacher now has available a number of known words that can be used for the development of specific reading skills. Children move into a more formal reading instruction process. It must be kept in mind that reading and reading instruction are different processes. Even at this stage, however, there probably will continue to be a need to use the language chart for a time until the mechanics are better integrated.

The Reading Chart

Once a chart has been prepared it should be used as is any other printed matter in directed reading activity instruction. This implies:

- a motivational phase involving needs assessment of the material and the children

- guided silent reading
- comprehension check and vocabulary development
- rereading when appropriate and necessary
- follow-up activities

The teacher has material in which the concepts, language, and organization were developed directly from the children. Therefore, why a needs assessment? The goals of the instruction may require different concepts, vocabulary, and organizational factors than those originally generated from the pupils. When this is true, the entire directed reading activity procedure should be followed.

To be effective as reading material, the reading chart must be well organized. To facilitate learning, repetition is a fundamental requirement. The basal reader attempts to do this by repeating a number of words through a number of different stories. The reading chart can generate repetition through varied usage. Therefore, a separate program must be developed that allows for repetition but precludes boredom. This is best accomplished with a five-day schedule:

- First day: introduction of the stimulus, development of concepts and vocabulary, and discussion of wording.
- Second day: review of previous day and writing of the chart; possible first teacher reading and rereading.
- Third day: first reading of chart for critical evaluation of language, sentence structure, etc.; frequent rereadings.
- Fourth day: purposeful rereading for word attack skills and repetition for sight vocabulary development.
- Fifth day: purposeful rereading for factual recall and inferential thinking.

This procedure provides the children with the opportunity for many rereadings to foster retention while developing specific skills or abilities that the teacher perceived as necessary. The specific goals of days three, four, and five should be determined by the teacher during the evaluations. For children with pronounced problems the schedule can be extended to seven days to allow greater repetition of vocabulary as well as intensified instruction on specific needs.

After seven days, however, it probably is better to develop another chart. Even with good, varied instruction, most children are ready to move on to a new stimulus or interest.

The initial chart should be stored in an accessible place. As other charts are completed, earlier ones should be reviewed and follow-up activities should require their use. This facilitates recall and application, both of which are vital to success.

Individual Charts

When a modified word learning procedure is used with language experience, the procedures are basically the same. The problem with sight vocabulary is less pressing since strictly auditory-visual learning is not required. However, all of the other facets described are appropriate. (See Appendix 6-D on writing.) The need for reviewing material cannot be overemphasized for learning disabled children, gifted or otherwise.

THE ULTIMATE GOAL

The language experience approach should have as its ultimate goal the reading of books, articles, forms, etc. Therefore, the teacher must be aware of already prepared materials that can be used for reading instruction. If the children have developed a chart or two on a specific topic and are demonstrating sufficient mastery, reading from a text might be done next. Pupils prepared through use of the charts should find such reading successful and rewarding. The standard directed reading activity should be used since it is hoped that some new ideas and vocabulary will appear in the text (Betts, 1946). If that is not to be the case, the materials should not be used for instructional goals. They might be useful, however, for motivational effect. Children like to have a feeling of success when dealing with books.

If books are to be used for instructional purposes, the teacher should be sure the children learn something new. Reading as a means of gaining information and solving problems must be stressed. In such situations, the readability factors often are irrelevant since the children bring much information and language to the task. (See Appendix 6-F on remedial instruction materials.)

REFERENCES

Betts, E.A. *Foundations of reading instruction.* New York: The American Book Company, 1946.

Lamoreaux, L.A., & Lee, P.M. *Learning to read through experience.* New York: D. Appleton-Century Company, 1943.

Appendix 6-A

Integrative Instruction

Much of the instruction for children with learning problems is based on highly structured systems approaches. It is possible that such approaches have merit. It also is possible that any particular learned ability is more than the sum of the skills. There is no real guarantee that because children are taught to recognize supporting details in isolation and a topic sentence in isolation that when they deal with a paragraph they will be able to integrate these specific skills into the ability called paragraph analysis.

One of the major problems of gifted/learning disabled children concerns that integrative process, so it would seem that teaching independent skills may be of little consequence in aiding these pupils. The suggestion here is that instruction for these individuals requires the integration of all the language skills within a framework of immediate interest.

Most highly intelligent children have areas of strong interest and an intense background of experience. Sometimes such interests and backgrounds can reach the point of being nearly obsessive. Yet they can be helpful in instruction. It is paradoxical that in many learning disability efforts, a total skills program is provided with no credence given to the learner's strengths. The pupil therefore finds the program not even related to what the pupil considers important. This also takes from the instruction a major element of learning theory—going from the known to the unknown.

Contrary to many skills programs' rationales, the child does not need to know certain words but rather words that contain the appropriate percepts for the concept desired. Rocket and comet, if known, are as useful as run and can, if known, for specific skill development.

The integrative process begins with the learner's interest and uses all four language processes whenever appropriate. A sense of rapport must be developed between learner and instructor. The teacher should show an interest in the pupil's interest and provide an honest interaction concerning the ideas, vocabulary,

51

concepts, and skills involved. An instructor who has a relevant background should interact; where this background is limited, that factor should be admitted. That may provide the best place for starting instruction.

Instruction should begin when the learner is convinced that there is something to share with the teacher or with others. At that point the instructor needs to be aware of certain fundamental questions:

- Can the learner express what he or she wishes to convey in any form? The instructor should record in writing the information presented.
- Is more information required or clarification important? The instructor needs to have appropriate reference resources available; in such a situation it often is most advantageous to read the material to the learner. (See Appendix 6-B on directed listening activity.)
- Can the learner organize the material in a suitable form? This form ought to be in the paragraph style of a good informational text with well-stated topic sentences and clearly listed details. The internal organization of the paragraph must be stressed and the correct sequence of paragraphs emphasized. Once again, it is important for the instructor to write the responses. By using writing, rereading is carried out easily, revisions made readily, and immediate evaluation provided.
- Can the learner appreciate that with proper organization, new vocabulary might be appropriate? The instructor on rereadings should inquire whether (1) the material sounds like a text, (2) the words are accurate and precise, and (3) there are more appropriate words for the context.

During these four stages the instruction will be basically Socratic, questions and answers, with the teacher doing the writing and providing constant clues to the learner concerning areas of needs. The emphasis is on the organization and evaluation of ideas on the oral/aural level. For many gifted/learning disabled children this is an absolutely vital technique. Because of the rigidity in vocabulary and ideas and limited versatility, this constant give and take meets needs in these two problem areas, as noted in Chapter 2.

Appendix 6-B

A Directed Listening Activity

In a listening activity it is important that the learner have reasons to listen. It is vitally important for children with learning difficulties and excellent intelligence to improve their organized behavior. Earlier it was mentioned that they tended not to be versatile and often were unable to organize their data well. It is the responsibility of the teacher of the gifted/learning disabled to foster improved performance. In many cases, these children suffer from an inability to distinguish the important from the trivial or unimportant.

An important starting point in improving listening ability is the teacher's goal: can the instructor develop in a learner the desire to obtain facts or appropriate information? What is to be listened for should always be appropriate to a pupil's learning task. This means that the teacher must arouse an interest or need if the learner does not already have one.

Obviously, the best way to develop this desire to obtain facts is to use materials that the learner is interested in. The reason for listening is to obtain new information. The child must always be placed in the position of being required to demonstrate in some fashion that the goal has been attained.

Listening activities may be used with individuals or small groups. A listening activity about geology might proceed as follows:

> Teacher: We have spent quite a bit of time discussing, really arguing, about the most common metal. We have had lots of opinions. This material probably has the answer for us. I want you to listen carefully to what I read. Do you all know what we are listening for? (Teacher should check to be sure the purpose is retained.) As soon as you have the answer, raise your hand. Please do not call out the answer.

The teacher begins to read the material. If the learners have a history of inattentiveness, the instructor, before the answer is reached, may have to use a technique that some educational purists may frown upon:

Teacher: Let's wait a minute. Did I read the answer yet? By the way, what were you listening to find out?

At this point the pupils can demonstrate whether they have retained the purpose for listening. If not, the purpose can be redeveloped and the reading continued. If the purpose has been retained, the children can be praised and the task continued.

Purists might complain that continuity has been destroyed. The point has little validity for two reasons:

1. If the purpose was forgotten, continuity is unimportant; if remembered, the continuity will follow.
2. The attitude of listening for comprehension initially is more important than the continuity of ideas. Nearly all children need help with listening but the gifted/learning disabled may require even more assistance since they are so often bored and frustrated at the same time.

It is vitally important to help the children implement the listening task on at least two levels: (1) they must process the language and the ideas it conveys; and (2) they must keep in mind the purpose for listening while they are listening; gifted/LD children often seem to lack this versatility and it needs to be cultivated.

Once the learners indicate that the goal has been reached, the teacher continues:

Teacher: You say you have the answer but what was your purpose? Good! Now what was the answer? Do you all agree?

If there is not total agreement, the teacher should restate the purpose and reread a few sentences before the answer appears or may reread the paragraph containing the answer. At this time, if a child or two is having trouble, the teacher should ask members of the group to explain how they arrived at the answer. If no peers are available, the teacher should demonstrate the thinking.

What follows next depends on the purpose that was developed. If the answer was strictly factual, then the teacher has no right to go back and question for information that was presented before the answer was delivered. To do so would once again do a great injustice to the gifted/LD children. Once again, they cannot anticipate the demands of teachers.

It is important to note that the purpose for listening gives direction to the learning. Gifted children often need to develop structure. If the purpose was inferential, the teacher has a right, possibly a responsibility, to ascertain whether any of the material presented prior to the answer has been retained. There is a real reason to suspect so. If the child uses the purpose well, there is a constant need to evaluate the material against the purpose. This constant evaluation should have provided information that the learner could recall even though it had no direct bearing on the purpose.

To be a good listener, the pupils eventually must begin to organize verbal data in light of what has been said and what might be said. That is why in a listening activity it is vital that gifted/LD pupils learn to use inferential purpose as soon as possible. As the first of the language abilities, it often is their only real beginning point. When listening is used poorly, it is almost a certainty that reading also will be poor. That statement may not be true of gifted children with no learning problems. Gifted pupils on a strictly egocentric basis "would rather do it myself." This is seldom true of learning problem children.

When the first purpose has been achieved, the teacher may continue the activity or stop. This decision should be based on whether or not the pupils have acquired appropriate information or merely supportive data. Of greater consequence is the decision concerning their ability to go on profitably. It is better to stop and, at the next meeting, start up after a short review than to proceed and put the child in a failure situation.

Whatever the decision, when the actual reading and discussions are finished, this activity needs to be followed up. Types of follow-ups might include:

- reading an easier book on the same topic and verifying the information listened to
- deciding on crucial words from the listening activity and learning them, using a word-learning technique, as in Appendix 6-C
- preparing an illustration, with labels if appropriate
- rewriting the information obtained when possible
- preparing questions that might need to be answered because of the information presented
- using audiovisual materials to supplement the materials read

The purposes of the listening activity are of special interest to the teacher. It was noted earlier that the purposes give direction to the learning. They permit the child to know what it is the instructor wants done or discovered. The purposes should be the means for the pupils to learn the knowns, or percepts, that will be necessary for them to develop the unknowns, or concepts, that the teacher believes are worthwhile for the children's well-being.

The instructor must know which concepts are to be developed and help the children acquire the appropriate percepts. This is the teacher's role. If learning is active, then teaching also must be active. Teachers must make decisions about the direction and rate of pupils' learning. Teachers must be even more active and direct with gifted/LD children, since in most cases the children's problem is that they lack these behaviors. The teachers must assume this burden until the pupils can.

Appendix 6-C

A Modified Fernald Procedure for Word Learning

Before this procedure is discussed in detail, a basic educational understanding must be developed and understood. This modification of the basic Fernald Procedure is not a methodology for teaching reading. In contrast to other multisensory approaches, this procedure is designed to help individuals learn words in a systematic way and eventually to be able to do so as an independent activity. The hoped-for outcome is little or no need for a teacher. It is a technique that can be used as long as a person needs to learn words. In a very real sense it is an effort to create independence in learning. This procedure essentially is a remedial technique for learning to read, but aspects and adaptations are very useful for developmental spelling and remedial writing, including remedial spelling.

The Fernald Procedure is a multisensory approach to learning words (Fernald, 1943). Basically, four, three, or two senses can be brought to bear on the learning task. The first two senses are those usually employed in all reading—visual and auditory (V-A). Learners see the words and hear the sound appropriate for them. This, then, is conventional visual-auditory learning.

The learners may look at the word and hear it while looking and then, while looking at the printed form, say the word. The kinesthetic (K), or movement, senses are then introduced. The movement is of the mouth, tongue, lips, etc. In effect this is V-A learning and V-K learning. This is called visual-auditory-kinesthetic learning (V-A-K).

If need be the pupils can look at and hear the word (V-A), look at and say the word (V-K), then look at-hear-say and feel the word. They can trace it with their fingers and feel the different textures through the tactile sense (T). While the child traces the word, if it is done properly, more kinesthetic learning is provided because of the movement of the arms. Therefore, the learning becomes visual-auditory-kinesthetic-tactile (V-A-K-T).

When the original procedure was analyzed later, it was recognized that tactile without kinesthetic learning was a nearly impossible procedure. Therefore, the

56

term haptic (H) was introduced. It indicates kinesthetic-tactile learning as an entity. The literature on remedial learning often uses V-A-H. This is nothing other than a restatement in more precise terms of V-A-K-T.

This modified procedure has certain premises:

- It is basically habilitative in nature.
- The learnings are basically gestalt, dealing with wholes before parts.
- Syllabic recognition and use is more helpful than single letter-sound correspondence.
- Analysis is more useful in word attack than is synthesis.

Certain essential materials are required for this technique:

- a dictionary at the learner's level, clearly written, with readable syllabication and varied meanings
- strips of newsprint, 4″ × 11″ to 12″, of poor quality (rough texture) for tracing
- large black crayons
- lined tablet and pencils
- shoebox
- anecdotal record sheets (described later)

INTRODUCING THE CONCEPT

After some rapport has been built, the teacher informs the pupils that there is a technique that will be successful for learning words. It is important to maintain a positive attitude. Learning should be emphasized.

It also must be explained that the technique must be mastered to be successful and that such mastery takes time. The instructor must be sure the learners appreciate this point so that initial discouragement does not set in. It should be emphasized that this probably is a new way of learning and at times the pupils will falter but that, with persistence, success will come.

INTRODUCING THE TECHNIQUE

The teacher should ascertain whether there is a word any learner has not been able to master in reading or writing. If the learners offer nothing (and many remain silent), any useful word may be suggested: the month, day, address, pupil's name, teacher's name, etc., as a beginning. It is important that learners understand that this technique can be used to comprehend and express their own personal ideas or interests. This is extremely important for the gifted/learning disabled since their interests and ideas have been subordinated to curriculum demands so often.

After the word has been selected, the following routine is *always* followed when the teacher is involved in the learning process:

1. "What does the word mean?" The teacher should accept an appropriate answer but should not press for semantic variation at this time since it can cause confusion.
2. "How many syllables, or parts, does it have?" The instructor should accept whatever the child offers but must remember the response, perhaps jotting down a note on it.
3. "Let's check the dictionary and see if you were correct." The teacher opens the dictionary to the appropriate section and locates the word.
4. The teacher points out the word to the child, verifies the meaning, and checks both the syllabication in print and respelling for pronunciation. If the pupil is correct about the syllables, the teacher makes a positive comment; if incorrect, the teacher says: "The word does not have _____ syllables. It has _____ syllables. Listen and I will say it for you." The teacher then should say the word clearly and slowly but should not drag out and distort the syllables.
5. The instructor again points out the word in the dictionary and says the syllables clearly.

At this point, the tracing slips are needed.

It usually is helpful to work with the child at a table. This provides space where books, boxes, and recording sheets, papers, etc., can be placed in an orderly, useful manner. Since the teacher needs to enter information on the anecdotal recording sheet, if the teacher is right-handed it is easier to work if the child sits to the instructor's left; the reverse is appropriate for left-handers.

The teacher writes the word on a tracing slip with the large black crayon. Before explaining how to write the word, the instructor will find certain physical procedures helpful. The teacher should:

1. slant the tracing slip so it is parallel to the child's eyes (it must be remembered that the word is being written for the child, not the teacher, to see)
2. hold the bottom of the tracing slip with the four fingers of the nonwriting hand; five or six tracing slips held together prevent slipping
3. hold the crayon extended by thumb, index, and middle fingers, rather straight, not in the position for gripping a pencil

In this way, the child will be able to see the word clearly as it is written. Writing is done using a cursive form. The teacher should:

1. say the whole word clearly and distinctly
2. start writing it syllable by syllable, saying each one normally and distinctly as it is being written
3. write the final syllable, then again say the whole word clearly and distinctly and dot "i's" and cross "t's," always left to right

For the word winter, this procedure would be:

"winter" = winter
"win" = win
"ter" = ter
"winter" = winter

The correct pronunciation of the syllable always is made as soon as the first stroke of the syllable is started. In this manner, the child receives visual and auditory input for the required word and its appropriate syllables.

Once the word is on the tracing slip correctly, the teacher then demonstrates to the child how to learn the word. The teacher:

1. Says "Watch what I do with this word because I want you to do the same thing."
2. Traces the word exactly as it was written, with the index and middle fingers joined as a type of stylus.
3. Places fingers on the beginning of the word and says it.
4. Says each syllable as it is started and follows the crayon with the fingers.
5. Dots "i" and "j" and crosses "t," always from left to right, then says the whole word again; if there are twin "t's," they are crossed individually from left to right.

When the word is checked in the dictionary, the lettering and the syllabication should be noted. This becomes a problem with a large number of words since visual and auditory coordination usually are not required but with this word-learning procedure this interaction is essential.

For example, the word winter provides no trouble. In the dictionary used (*Webster's* , 1976), it is win = "win," ter = "ter." What can be said about the word double? It is a little different: dou = "doub," ble = "el." When writing it for the child, the teacher says, double; dou = "doub," ble = "el." When tracing it, the teacher follows the same procedure and when the child does so, the correct procedure must be followed.

If some children have trouble (trou = "troub," etc.) with double or similar words, the teacher might want to underline the syllables to force the attention to the print while saying it precisely.

Once the word is written correctly and demonstrated by the teacher on the tracing slip, the following procedure should be followed:

1. The child traces the word as often as necessary until the learner feels it can be written as traced. If an error in tracing occurs, the teacher stops the child and demonstrates the correct procedure. This may have to be repeated.
2. The child then attempts to write the word exactly as traced, using a pencil on the back of a tracing slip held lengthwise.

At that point, there are two alternatives: correct or incorrect writing. If the writing is exactly correct in terms of both letter formation and sequence and of pronunciation, the child is asked to check the writing against the correct form on the front of the tracing slip. This provides, of course, another learning experience. Once it is checked, the child is told to write it again exactly the same way, inserting the word, again written totally correctly, into the article, story, form, etc., in which the word was required. All of this should be entered on the anecdotal record sheet. (See Appendix 6-E on that subject.)

If an error has occurred in writing, the procedure should be as follows:

1. The teacher stops the child immediately, the error is covered with another tracing slip, and the type of error is noted on the anecdotal record sheet.
2. The teacher then tells the child to watch as the tracing of the word is demonstrated again.
3. The teacher asks the child if the word needs to be traced again and encourages the pupil to do so as often as it is needed.
4. The child then attempts to write the word again as in the previous procedure. All preceding attempts, right or wrong, are covered up.

When the child is correct, the word is inserted into the appropriate material and the teacher continues dictating until the next error occurs, when the procedure is followed again.

THE INTRODUCTORY STAGE

At the laboratory school of the reading clinic of Temple University (Johnson & Kress, 1966) where this modification of the Fernald Procedure evolved and has been used with great success, the preceding routine is titled the *introductory stage*. Its real purpose is to have the child learn the technique. It is characterized by teacher demonstration.

In a short time, the child usually tells the teacher that demonstration no longer is necessary. The pupil feels confident that after the teacher writes the word on the slip there will be no trouble in doing the tracing.

STAGE 1

As soon as that happens, the child has moved into *stage 1*. The only difference between the introductory and first stages is that in the latter, the teacher no longer traces the word before the child tries it.

Two cautions are necessary here. First, some children with severe learning problems, no matter how intelligent they may be, are fearful of striking out on their own. After a few days they should be encouraged to do so. Second, most children are in two stages at the same time. They may feel a need for demonstration on one word, often a long one, but feel perfectly secure to go ahead with tracing on another. This is not a problem; it is the usual way for most children.

Children without associative learning problems often go through both of these stages quickly.

STAGE 2

When a child is operating in stage 1 successfully, the next change occurs. After looking at the tracing slip as written by the teacher, the child will feel that there is no need for tracing. This is *stage 2*. The teacher then proceeds as follows:

> Good! Let me show you how I want you to learn this word. First, look at the whole word and say it correctly. Next, look at each syllable. As you look at it, say it. Now look at the whole word again and say it. Do this until you think you can write it exactly as we did when tracing.

The child, if learning "winter," would say,

"winter" = winter
"win" = win
"ter" = ter
"winter" = winter

This procedure is repeated until the child feels capable of writing on the back of the tracing slip as previously. (The recording is different for this stage, as noted in Appendix 6-E since no demonstration or tracing marks are required.)

Tracing slips still are used even though the child has moved into stage 2 since some words probably will still need to be traced. The transition from stage to stage usually is smooth; seldom do children hop abruptly from one to the next. Tracing slips can be used at any stage.

Once a child is operating at stage 2 consistently, the tracing slip is dropped and the use of a 3" × 5" or 4" × 6" file card is introduced. At this point, the teacher writes the word with a pencil in large cursive letters on the front of the card, with the card in a horizontal position. The child writes on the back, with the card in a vertical position. The same procedure for precision in the task, correctness in reproduction, and exactness in the routine still is required.

STAGE 3

Later, when the teacher points out a word in the dictionary, the child will comment that the teacher does not need to write it out. This is transition into *stage 3*. The teacher next proceeds as follows:

> Good! Since I do not have to write it for you, let me show you how I want
> you to learn it.
> Look at the word in the dictionary. Say it.
> Look at each syllable and say it.
> Then look at the whole word again and say it.
> Do this until you think you can write it.

At this point, the procedure for the child changes. When the pupil writes the word, it is on the back of the card. After this has been done twice correctly, it must be written again correctly in the middle on the front of the card as a file copy. Therefore, in stage 3, as opposed to the other stages, there must be three consecutive correct reproductions. An error in any of these requires the child to begin anew. This third reproduction obviously provides enhanced reinforcement kinesthetically.

STAGE 4

Stage 4 of the technique, which is not really encouraged for students with associative learning problems, is studying the word from the dictionary as in stages 2 and 3 but then inserting it into a context immediately. It is strictly auditory-visual learning.

By the end of each day's instruction, the teacher will have listed on the anecdotal record sheet the words learned during that session. These words then become the basis for reinforcement, enrichment, and application activities.

REFERENCES FOR APPENDIX 6-C

Fernald, G.M. *Remedial techniques in basic school subjects*. New York: McGraw-Hill Book Company, Inc., 1943.

Johnson, M.S., & Kress, R.A. *Eliminating word-learning problems in reading disability cases*. Philadelphia: Temple University Reading Clinic, 1966.

Webster's new world dictionary. Englewood Cliffs, N.J.: Prentice-Hall, Inc., 1976.

Appendix 6-D

The Writing Activity

Once the teacher has prepared the composition, the actual pupil writing should begin. However, it must be reemphasized here: the entire oral/aural activity should have dealt with vocabulary, varied sentence structure, paragraphing, grammar, syntax, etc. By this time the teacher should have the best possible form from which the learner can work.

DICTATION AND WRITING

The process initially involves the teacher's dictation of the material as the learner writes it down. Usually the procedure is as follows:

> Teacher: Now we are ready for writing. Do you have all of your materials? [See Appendix 6-C, on the modified Fernald Procedure.] Now let me read you the title and the first paragraph.

The learner begins to write, starting with the title, if there is one. The teacher must note that everything is done correctly—title and first word of sentence capitalized, capitalization accurate, etc. If an error occurs, the teacher stops the writing and asks if it can be corrected. In the case of a spelling error, the teacher proceeds with the modified word-learning procedure; if it is a punctuation mistake, it is discussed and the correct form taught immediately. The type of error should be noted on the anecdotal record form so that more intensive instruction can be given later. The learner then works through the paragraphs for the instructional time allotted. This time may vary from 20 to 45 minutes, depending on administrative circumstances and the learner's ability to stay on task.

At the end of the time, the instructor must deal with two immediate concerns: What does the learner do now? What does the teacher do with the child's written material?

If there is any real truth in learning theory, it is necessary to accept the concept that the learner must do something to learn. Learning is an active, not a passive, activity. This concept also is necessary for a teacher's effective functioning with a class. Each learner must be able to do something academically important alone or with minimal help. The basic need is a worthwhile follow-up activity. In many respects for children with learning difficulties, these activities may well be the most significant procedure a teacher uses.

To be totally effective, three aspects of learning must be addressed:

1. retention: providing enough repetition of things taught most recently
2. recall: relating new learning to past learning
3. application: keeping learnings alive through usage

Therefore, any follow-up activity should address these three issues. The activity might involve listening and/or viewing but it should always include some type of motor activity, especially writing.

For example, in the course of a day's writing a child interested in geology learns the following words: rocks, sedimentary, precipitates, and pebbles. The teacher knows the child tends to be rigid in vocabulary usage so work on semantic variation is indicated.

The word "rocks" could be useful immediately. The instructor might prepare an activity in which "rocks" takes on different meanings:

> *Directions:* Put *rocks* into all blanks where it is right. If you cannot put rocks in the blank, put an X.
> The wave _____ the boat.
> The mother _____ the baby to sleep.
> The man finds the _____ in the sky.

If work on using commas in a series were at issue, the following activity can be helpful:

> *Directions:* Put commas in all the places where they should go.
> Stones pebbles rocks and shells may be precipitates.
> Wind waves and man rock the boats.
> Some metals that run through rocks are gold copper and silver.

Extended versions of these activities can be a part of the follow-up. If the child also is having difficulty with analogies and that has been a subject of work by the teacher, the instructor could use some analogies with past information and present learning:

Directions: Fill in the blanks below from words you have learned. You may use your file box.

Smoke is to rise as rain is to _____.

Salt is to water as gold is to _____.

Lava is to igneous as sandstone is to _____.

The child may have had a history of difficulty with capitalization. The following activity could provide useful practice and application:

Directions: Read the paragraph below. Some words need capital letters. Put capital letters on all words that need them.

the hot earth

the earth is very hot inside. sometimes lava comes out of the ground. lava is melted rock. inside the earth it is called magma.

With four examples such as these in an expanded form, children should be provided with independent activities of a worthwhile nature that require as much time as was spent in the direct teaching, if not more. This useful time for the students allows the teacher to work with other children on their identified needs. However, it must be noted that the teacher must have time to prepare these activities each day.

MATERIALS BECOME TEXT

What must be done with the child's handwritten material? It should be remembered that the activity is to be totally integrative of all four language areas. The handwritten material now is to be converted into a text for reading instruction. The teacher should keep in mind how functional this will be. The child will have the total background in concepts, vocabulary, and skills necessary for reading this material. This factor makes it ideal for teaching reading skills. However, it first must be developed for reading, which means transforming the handwritten material into print.

It is suggested that the following procedures be used:

1. The material should be typed with large, clear print in manuscript form (with carbon copy). The typing must be an exact copy of the child's work.
2. When this is completed, the original should be turned face to face with the carbon. The learned words are typed on the back of the original in a column that does not intrude into the typed area of the carbon. This should produce one original text with a list of learned words on the back and a carbon copy with the text and the column of learned words on the front (Figure 6-D-1). The use of this material is discussed later.

Figure 6-D-1 Transferring Child's Material—First Day

(original)

My Turtle

My turtle is nine weeks old.

(carbon)

My Turtle

My turtle is nine weeks old.

F   U   C

My
Turtle
nine
weeks
old

Key: F = Flash, sight vocabulary. U = Untimed, application of attack skills in isolation.
C = Context, recognition of word in original setting.

---

3. Each day as new material is developed, the same procedure is followed by adding it to the original (Figure 6-D-2). The typed original text becomes longer with a series of columns of learned words but the carbon copy each day contains only the one day's writing and the list of that day's learned words.

4. This procedure is followed until the text of the child's written copy of the dictated material appears intact on the original (Figure 6-D-3).

These daily typed materials are used to measure short-term retention, usually 24 hours. The retention is measured in three ways: (F) flash, sight vocabulary; (U)

Figure 6-D-2 Transferring Child's Material—Second Day

(original)

My Turtle

My turtle is nine weeks old. He eats lettuce,
hamburger

(carbon)

He eats lettuce,
hamburger

F   U   C

lettuce
My   hamburger
Turtle
nine
weeks
old

Key: F = Flash, sight vocabulary. U = Untimed, application of attack skills in isolation.
C = Context, recognition of word in original setting.

---

untimed, application of attack skills in isolation; and (C) context, recognition of the word in its original setting. If at any point the child does not make a response, the letter "O" (for omission) is inserted in the appropriate space.

The following procedure should be used when a writing activity is initiated:

1. Using the words on the back of the original for yesterday's writing, flash the word tachistoscopically to the child. If the child calls the word correctly, move to the next word. No marks are made on the carbon under F or U when the answer is correct.

Figure 6-D-3 Transferring Child's Material—Third Day

(original)

My Turtle

My turtle is nine weeks old. He eats lettuce,
hamburger and bugs. He eats in the water. I feed him
meat on a straw.

(carbon)

and bugs. He eats in the water. I feed him
meat on a straw.

	lettuce		F	U	C
My	hamburger	water			
Turtle		feed			
nine		meat			
weeks		straw			
old					

Key: F = Flash, sight vocabulary. U = Untimed, application of attack skills in isolation.
C = Context, recognition of word in original setting.

---

2. If the child miscalls the word, ask the child to look at it and apply word attack skills. While the child is looking at the word, record the error under F. It should be recorded verbatim since this can help identify the type of mistake.
3. If the child then calls the word correctly, place a check-mark under the U to indicate an accurate response. If the child still miscalls the word, the error is recorded verbatim.
4. Once all the words have been dealt with in isolation, tell the child to read the material silently. Set a purpose for the reading. Then ask the child to read the

material aloud. Any word that is read correctly in context, but was not read correctly in flash (F) or untimed (U), is noted on the carbon under context (C).

5. A percentage of correctness is then determined for each aspect. Scores are given only for correct responses in flash. On the untimed, all correct answers on flash and the untimed corrections are counted together. For context, all other correct responses and knowns in context are combined to make the score. The percentage is obtained by dividing the number of correct responses by the number possible. Figure 6-D-4 is an example of such scoring.

Figure 6-D-4 Examples of Scoring

	F	U	C
My			
Turtle			
nine			
weeks			
old			
My	F	U	C
Turtle			
nine			
weeks			
old			
lettuce	F	U	C
hamburger			
lettuce	F	U	C
hamburger			
water	F	U	C
feed			
meat			
straw			

Key: F = Flash, sight vocabulary. U = Untimed, application of attack skills in isolation. C = Context, recognition of word in original setting. √ = correct response. O = omission (no response).

Appendix 6-E

Recordkeeping and Daily Anecdotal Record Sheet

The daily anecdotal record sheet is a vital component of the remediation program. It serves a number of important functions:

- It provides structure for the learner since it must be filled out at the beginning of the instructional segment and must be maintained in an orderly fashion throughout.
- It provides a running account of the program, progress or lack thereof, and documentable changes, accumulated over a week, a month, or a year. It also produces excellent documentation of program consistency and adherence to stated objectives.
- It becomes the basis for initial word learning since the child also must fill out part of it. The month of the year, academic terms, and names all are necessary items to be learned.

Each day each child is given a record sheet. (Figure 6-E-1 is an example of such a sheet with information filled in.) For cost-effective purposes it could be reproduced front and back and therefore be used for two days. The three blanks at the top should always be filled out: child's name; teacher's name; and month, day, and year. The month always should be written, not numbered. Any such facts that are not known should be learned by the modified Fernald Procedure.

The two left-hand columns, time and activities, are the child's responsibilities. Time can be written as 9:00, etc. This is extremely important for learning disabled children who have time concept difficulties. Clock reading and time structures can be enhanced because of the consistency and repetition of the sheet. Activities are scheduled procedures that need to be written out. Words such as opening, reading, arithmetic, recess, science, etc., usually appear in this column. Therefore, when the student fills out the sheet correctly, an observer would know what time an activity was initiated and when the next one followed. Once again, this is an excellent source for word learning.

71

The last two columns, Comments and Word Learning, are filled in by the teacher. The comments column should contain short anecdotal notes about behavior—satisfactory or unsatisfactory. If possible, it should be written beside the activity in which it was observed. It also is the place to note learning errors. This notation is extremely important during word learning. A useful system is for the teacher to note the error, then write a slash, then what was expected. A small *r* or *w* indicates whether it was a reading or writing error. For example, house/horse (*r*) would indicate the substitution of house for horse in reading. In writing, it would be hou-/horse (*w*). This indicates that as soon as the teacher saw the incorrect vowel, the writing was stopped. With this type of information, the dynamics of skills difficulties become apparent in a real way without the artificiality of tests or inventories.

The word learning column records the child's performance in using the modified Fernald Procedure. Certain basic recording symbols were developed at the laboratory school of the Reading Clinic at Temple University for use with the procedure. They have proved to facilitate understanding of written records. The symbols are:

d = demonstration
/ = accurate tracing
/\ = faulty tracing
√ = correct reproduction
√\ = incorrect reproduction

As the child moves through the procedure, fewer of the symbols are needed. For the introductory or demonstration stage, all five probably will be used. Each demonstration, tracing, or reproduction is noted. At stage 1, no demonstrations are given, so that symbol does not appear. At stages 2 and 3, no tracing is done, so those symbols disappear. Eventually only the correct or incorrect check is used.

When children are in transition from the introductory level to stage 1, and from stage 1 to stage 2, the symbols clearly indicate the stage of operation. This is not true from stage 2 to stage 3; therefore, a small 2 or 3 is noted in front of the word learned to indicate the level of operation.

The filled-in daily anecdotal record sheet contains situations rather unlikely to have occurred; it is used simply to illustrate the marking system. The words and their symbols mean the following:

eggs: two demonstrations; two faulty tracings; two more demonstrations; two correct tracings; a correct, then an incorrect, reproduction; another demonstration; three correct tracings; and finally, two correct reproductions. The child is in the introductory or demonstration stage.

scum: two demonstrations, two correct tracings, a faulty one, and two correct reproductions.

fish: two correct tracings, a faulty one, two correct tracings, then two correct reproductions. The child is in stage 1.

tadpole: three correct tracings and two correct reproductions.

toes: two faulty reproductions, a correct reproduction, a faulty reproduction, then two correct reproductions. The child is in stage 2.

jump: a faulty reproduction, then two correct reproductions.

bugs: two correct reproductions. The child is in stage 3.

Figure 6-E-1 Example of a Filled-In Daily Record Sheet

Daily Record Sheet

Name: *Billy Smith*   Date: *May 2, 1982*

Teacher: *Mrs. Harris*

Time	Activities	Comments	Word Learning
9:00	Opening	Billy did not cry coming to school today. He sulked a little during the pledge of Allegiance.	
9:05	Reading Bats in Caves	Likes this story. Very attentive. Calls out too often.	
9:30	Writing	fire/flames (R) dark/damp (R) Is still working on frog article.	egg d/// ✓✓ scum dd // ✓✓ fish // ^ // ✓✓ tadpole /// ✓✓ (2) toes ✓✓ ✓^✓✓ (3) jump ✓ ✓✓ (4) bugs ✓✓
10:00 10:10 10:40	Recess Follow-up I. R.		

Key: d = Demonstrating. / = Accurate tracing. ^ = Faulty tracing. ✓ = Correct reproduction. ✓^ = Incorrect reproduction. (2) and (3) = Stage of operation.

Appendix 6-F

Materials for Remedial Instruction

A remedial program should have as its first goal the dispelling of ignorance. The question always should be, "What do you want the child to know?" not, "What do you want the child to do?" Once it has been determined what the child should know, then the doing or skills aspects become self-evident.

It is important for a student to obtain data because reading is a data retrieval process. All students should have a background in science, social studies, health, and safety and survival skills. Since learning disabled youths are a part of all children, then this must be true of them also. Gifted children in many cases need to have their horizons broadened and new interests spurred. They must be exposed to a variety of concepts and curriculum areas.

Instructional materials for the gifted/learning disabled child should as much as possible be content oriented. That is, they should involve those areas in which data is the main component, rather than fictionalized experiences. Because of the intense interests of many of these children it is vital that these materials be made available. This is true for all age levels. The children often have specific concepts and vocabulary that permit access to materials that might appear too difficult from a readability standpoint. Sciences of all types, hobbies, construction, etc., offer excellent materials for reading instruction for these children.

The reader may wonder why literary materials were excluded from the suggestions above. Gifted/learning disabled children often find that the fictional works offered at their independent and instructional reading levels are boring. However, this does not mean that literature should not be a part of their lives. It can be made available to them through listening activities, since they cannot use the reading process to avail themselves of appropriate materials. Formalized listening activities should be a regular part of the educational program. This is an excellent way to expand the interests of the group of children receiving instruction.

It is difficult to have a program developing concepts with children when the concepts are based on highly individualized past experiences. The concepts (inferences) based on such experiences are opinions or prejudices and vary from individual to individual. What is right or wrong, good or bad, happy or sad, considerate or stupid is determined by the person's background. Education is society's way of providing children with facts and helping them develop concepts of the world. No wonder children are confused, since emotions and feelings are unique to each individual. However, water boils at 212°F at sea level for everyone.

The remedial program suggested here begins with a curriculum base. The area to be examined should be determined by children's interests. Rocks, rockets, animals, or dinosaurs cause no problem since the material is written in English and the skills patterns are the same.

A language experience approach that involves the language and ideas of the child is an important technique. The teacher's goal is to develop the necessary sight vocabulary from which the children can develop their skills. The language experience approach produces the necessary repetition for retention to occur and does so in a sensible, not a rote, fashion. Familiarity and understanding are the elements necessary for satisfactory recall.

Parents must be sure to display an interest in developing concepts. In the home, all things should be talked about. In the kitchen, the parents should speak of and have the child respond to spatula, slotted spoon, saucepan, broiler, etc. Once verbal command is demonstrated, games involving these words can be developed, putting the word on the correct object, finding the printed word for a definition, and running through the words in isolation as a final step.

In this procedure children also are building a reservoir of knowledge and information. It is these data that can be so important to the development of self-esteem. It is vital for a child to be able to demonstrate to family and peers information and ideas that they might not have. "I know the name of the highest mountain in the world. Do you?" is often the unfolding of a sense of self-worth.

For gifted/learning disabled children, the language experience using content materials means that they will not be subjected to elements designed for children of an earlier age or interest level. The concept of being held to a reader level is negated. Instead, skills development and understandings can be maintained at the children's development level so they can learn material appropriate to their intelligence and interests.

One problem with the concept of interests is that parents and teachers tend to make decisions about what interests are appropriate for the children. They should encourage the learner's own interests; the imposing of interests never has worked. When the language experience approach is used correctly, interests develop, producing a need for information and ideas. In some cases, the materials may be beyond the learners' measured reading abilities; these can be read and explained to them. In other cases, because they have developed a background in a particular area, the children read materials that are above their level.

There are a number of obvious adjustments that the school and remedial teachers must make to develop such a program:

- The school (principal, superintendent, school board) must accept different management principles, that is, the setting of short-range goals. Evaluations cannot be based on grade level or reader level but on skills development. This means the acceptance of criterion-referenced inventories and procedures for evaluation of progress.
- The teacher should be allowed to use materials other than those prescribed by grade or achievement level.
- Teacher or school reports to parents should be based on the acquisition of skills rather than on subjective evaluation by grade.
- The remedial teacher and the classroom teacher should be required to cooperate and plan for the good of the child and time must be provided for them to do such planning.

These adjustments would have to be made, whether or not the child was mainstreamed. Too frequently, mainstreaming appears to have been removed from its fundamental purpose of providing the least restrictive environment. Mainstreaming offers the best hope in the socialization and the psychological well-being of handicapped learners. When it is used in place of growth in the process aspects of the teaching-learning area there appears to be real doubt that such an outcome could be forthcoming. Individual needs must be addressed in these areas.

Teachers using a content approach need to be more versatile in pedagogical skills and techniques. The important aspect they should keep in mind is that there is no one way or best way to learn to read. They must understand that a procedure that is effective for a normal 7-year-old may not be useful for a gifted 12-year-old.

Materials can be a problem and often are given as a reason for not using a content approach to remedial instruction. However, lack of material is not a sound reason for not teaching through content. There are three types of content materials that can be used in this approach:

1. commercially prepared (often too difficult to begin the program)
2. child-prepared language experience approach charts and exercises
3. adult-prepared materials designed by a teacher, aide, or volunteer to meet specific curriculum and skills goals

Child-prepared and adult-prepared materials should not become ends in themselves. The teacher's goal must be student use of prepared texts. The texts might be books, magazines, articles, flyers, etc., but they should demand of the users the techniques that successful readers employ. Programs that rely wholly on materials adjusted to meet reading problems (or levels) fail because learning disabled children will not have such materials handed to them forever. The instruction should focus on normally presented materials. As the children develop concepts and vocabulary and as their sight vocabularies increase, the teacher can develop the appropriate process skills. When these two components—sight vocabulary and word attack skills—are comprehended, the children should begin to use commercially prepared materials.

The role of parents in a content reading program for gifted/learning disabled children is important in some fundamental ways:

- They must make an honest attempt to support the concept with their children; they should delight in the pupils' informational growth, not just their word-calling ability.
- They should encourage the school and teachers to help the children think, to use their abilities, to attack problems, and to become independent. Parents must recognize that, with help, a child can become inner directed, not outer directed and dependent.
- They should be interested in things. Parents should be willing to encourage interests in the children. Trips based on specific goals are more important than mere generalized sight-seeing jaunts—visiting the zoo to look at the snakes is far better than just visiting the zoo. This activity provides the concept for directed, purposeful behavior, not generalized random movement.

There is no implication here that such a program will develop "readers." It is very difficult for a child hurt by the reading process to ever "love to read." The emotional consequences of failure and lack of achievement are usually severe for these children. It is possible that the concept of developing a love for reading in these children is the reason that so many remedial programs fail. The goal of a content reading program is to help children use reading as the necessary tool that it is. If they can find delight in it, that is a bonus. The real goal is to have the child use reading as a process, successfully and without fear.

Appendix 6-G

Developmental, Remedial, and Adaptive Procedures

When dealing with learning problems, continuous assessments and evaluations are necessary. These are particularly important after an instructional program has been in effect for a reasonable period of time. The results of the assessments and evaluations provide guidelines for changes in instructional procedures.

Instructional procedures can be viewed from three different points of view:

1. Developmental: This includes all practices associated with regular instructional activities. There are no fundamental skills or process difficulties that preclude normal learning. Visual-auditory learning provides enough stimulation, and memory processes are at least adequate.
2. Remedial: This includes all practices that in effect provide learning through added stimulation or rigorously designed instructional processes. These may include multisensory learning approaches for added sensory stimulation or complex skills programs based on tight management principles.
3. Adaptive: This includes all practices that in effect bypass the developmental and remedial procedures. These practices could include the use of typewriters or tape recorders in place of writing, hand calculators for memory problems in mathematics, readers or peer tutors for reading disabilities, and microcomputers. The adaptive materials might be housed in a learning center, while some adaptive procedures should be permitted in the classroom.

The decision as to which one (if not all three) of these techniques is to be used is crucial for many learning disabled children. This is especially true for the gifted/learning disabled. The inability or reluctance of educators to permit or to employ various approaches to instruction has had a destructive effect on children with problems.

Children who can use developmental procedures should do so. These techniques are faster, more efficient, and less liable to bring derision upon the pupils. Interestingly, if they can use developmental procedures, they probably did not have a learning disability in the first place. In most such cases, the lack of achievement probably resulted from institutional retardation, i.e., programs insensitive to the children's processes. The pupils were forced into regimented instruction to which they could not adapt. If a different approach had been used, the problems would not have occurred. This may well be a major reason for the lack of academic achievement that now is called learning disability.

Remedial procedures should be used with nearly all learning disabled children who are labeled correctly. These procedures tend to be slower paced since greater child involvement is required and more elaborate reinforcement and enrichment activities must be provided. Appendixes 6-C, 6-D, 6-E, and 6-F in this text focus on remedial procedures. There are numerous texts on multisensory approaches to reading (Adamson & Adamson, 1979; Betts, 1946; Fernald, 1943; Wallace & Kauffman, 1973) and systems methods of various types are available commercially. Remedial procedures can work, enabling learning disabled children to function nearly normally.

However, there is one major problem. Schools and "remedial" programs have refused consistently to use remedial procedures. The most common reason offered for rejection is that these techniques are too slow and time consuming. The fact that the children require remedial procedures is not even understood. Many schools, and especially administrators, seem to feel that there must be a quick remedial program or a developmental program that also is remedial. The inconsistency and illogic of this position can only lead to further pain for all concerned. Remedial education must be an accepted practice. (See Chapters 17, 18, and 19.)

Adaptive procedures, though still relatively new for learning problems, are beginning to suffer the same fate as the remedial procedures in many schools. Educators and the public in general have no compunctions about supplying physically handicapped children with braces, hearing aids, crutches, etc., yet adaptive devices for the learning handicapped are considered to be wrong. Many schools do not allow children with mathematics handicaps or short-term memory problems to use hand calculators. Many children who "cannot do long division" actually can perform such calculations; what they cannot do is recall the number facts that make the division succeed. Some schools frown on the use of peer tutors to help with reading since it can make it difficult to evaluate the child for grading purposes. Success that could be generated academically is prohibited so schools can stress the scale of grades.

In a program for gifted/learning disabled children, the major emphasis should be on remedial procedures. Words and number facts can be learned using a modified Fernald Procedure. Elements that require short-term memory skills can be kept to a few items. It is better to learn three words or three number facts than to attempt six and learn none of them.

In many cases a direct request to the learner, "What could I do to help you with this?" often brings a very insightful response. Children often recognize their problems and may even have learned compensatory or adaptive behavior. Those who learned to count on their fingers because they could do it no other way are demonstrating adaptive techniques.

Few gifted/learning disabled children require a totally adaptive program. In most cases, remediation is sufficient. However, many of these children need adaptive techniques for specific elements, most commonly in written language. The typewriter and computer may be vital adaptive devices if used intelligently (see Appendix 6-H).

REFERENCES FOR APPENDIX 6-G

Adamson, W.C., & Adamson, M.S. *A handbook for specific learning disabilities*. New York: Gardner Press, 1979.

Betts, C.A. *Foundations of reading instruction*. New York: American Book Co., 1946.

Fernald, G. *Remedial techniques in basic school subjects*. New York: McGraw-Hill, 1943.

Wallace, G., & Kauffman, J.M. *Teaching children with learning problems*. Columbus, Ohio: C.E. Merrill, 1973.

Appendix 6-H

The Role of Computers

The age of the individual computer obviously has arrived. The effects of this electronic marvel are being felt nationwide and even worldwide, yet far too many schools and education programs pay little attention to this development. In the education of gifted/learning disabled children, the individual computer must be integrated as a necessary component of the instructional program. Computer literacy training can be started with first graders as well as middle school children.

Because of their intelligence, interests, and awareness, gifted children probably require more stimulation of ideas than their nongifted peers. For nondisabled gifted children, much of this stimulation can come from printed matter—books and magazines become important components of their development. However, with gifted/learning disabled children this is seldom the case. Printed materials, especially books, symbolize their unhappiness, low self-esteem, and failure. Yet to prosper, they also need stimulation. The individual computer offers an alternative.

Because a computer can supply information and ideas in various modes, it is useful for the gifted/learning disabled. The language emphasized can quickly become sight vocabulary because of the necessary repetitions. Graphics can be read and information obtained with a minimum of reading ability. In some situations a voice synthesizer can provide aural stimulation for the visual presentation.

Many of the simulations and games can provide intellectual challenge without requiring much reading or writing ability. Challenges that would be difficult to derive from a text or impossible to get from a teacher overburdened with other students can be obtained from a computer program. The computer's impersonal acceptance of their performance often is welcomed by children with learning problems who feel threatened by teachers' corrections. The computer seldom scolds, seldom is derogatory.

Gifted/learning children not only benefit from the instructional value of computer programs, they also take very readily to computer management procedures. They should be taught how to use the computer's switches, buttons, keys, discs, etc., as well as the language and art of programming itself. From recent experience it is evident that they can learn that language.

In 15 half-hour instructional periods during a practicum for gifted/learning disabled, 7- and 8-year-olds learned to use the computer well enough to begin rudimentary programs of materials of their own design. Finally, they should receive instruction on developing instructional programs for use by their peers or other children. The intellectual discipline of developing goals and following through with an orderly thought process is invaluable to them and could be for all achieving children.

Computers constitute an untapped resource for children with writing problems. Computers are consistent in word usage, reinforcement, and development of spelling. When a child fails to spell correctly, the computer can be programmed to simply stop. It does not chastise; it simply halts. Inconsistent use of language may well make a child's hour-long effort in programming useless. A few of these mishaps can stimulate the student to ensure precision.

For many children, the spelling errors noted so often on their papers in red pencil are not mistakes in the true sense of letter-by-letter sequencing. They are handwriting errors. Many gifted/learning disabled children correctly spell orally words that they miswrite. Taking the handwriting out of writing activities for many of these children brings about a totally different attitude.

Many of the advantages of computers can be obtained with a typewriter. However, the programming demands that are so important are not found in simple typing. A caution must be raised here. Whenever typing is involved, conventional touch typing tends to be recommended automatically. In many cases this is exactly the wrong procedure. Many learning disabled children have fine motor problems, and touch typing requires fine motor skills, so such a recommendation can negate what otherwise could be a very successful learning experience. Another failure has been added. Something that aroused the child's enthusiasm and desire is once again unavailable because of the disability. It is easy to understand the child's negative attitude and behavior if the cause is analyzed or investigated seriously.

When computer instruction begins, children who have demonstrated difficulties with fine motor skills should not receive touch typing. This problem can be discovered during writing tasks. These children should be taught how to type in "journalism" style, using the two index fingers. They should be permitted to use a hunt-and-peck system until they develop one of their own. Many adults who type in this fashion are just as efficient as conventional typists. A disability should not vitiate a task that could be compensated for by a perfectly acceptable different method.

Throughout this book the concept of bright children interacting with bright children has been stressed. As with most principles, there are instances where this concept must be modified. When using computers, two bright children working together may not be the best procedure. For teachers this seems more efficient, but it is probably not as effective as a single child on the computer at one time.

Because most gifted children, including learning disabled ones, tend to use divergent thinking they operate in different fashions. Their approaches to problems and ensuing solutions are quite individualistic. Since the computer by its nature must be treated consistently, two children operating differently cause trouble. As noted earlier, speed of reaction flexibility, etc., between two gifted children can be so different that friction develops. It is far better to allow one child a shorter period of time on the computer than to provide an extended time for two.

Those who see joint effort as a means of fostering interaction and cooperation should be aware that isolation and separation can develop far more easily. This is true in games and simulations as well as in learning activities. Games and simulations should be the only activities in which cooperative behavior is attempted. Even in this situation, care must be taken to partner children who have similar response patterns. Even though there may be two children with IQs of 140, if one is impetuous and the other plodding, the value of the program will disappear. There are many other activities in which cooperative behavior can be encouraged. The substantial value of the individual computer for gifted/learning disabled children can be dissipated by thoughtless use.

Appendix 6-I

Literacy and Its Varied Aspects

When working with children who have had great difficulty learning, a time arrives when some decisions must be made about what is to be learned. That decision is crucial since it ought to reflect an honest appraisal of what the child wants, needs, and is capable of. With many gifted/learning disabled children that determination often is affected by the counselor's recognition of the student's basic intelligence, which clouds the realities of the situation. Even though a child is highly intelligent, certain tasks or accomplishments may not be attainable at any given time.

Those involved in teaching the gifted/learning disabled, especially older children and youths, many times will have to resolve the dilemma of potential vs. possible.

As posited here, there are three basic types of literacy: literacy, functional literacy, and stratified literacy:

1. Literacy: the vocabulary and thinking/reading skills that allow an individual to use print materials for relaxation, enjoyment, self-improvement, and intellectual enlightenment.
2. Functional Literacy: the vocabulary and thinking/reading skills that allow a person to deal successfully with routine print materials of daily living such as road signs, forms, machine directions, directories, etc.
3. Stratified Literacy: the vocabulary and thinking/reading skills that apply directly to a specific area, profession, trade, etc. It includes jargon and technical vocabulary as well as specific reading skills such as diagram reading, following directions, organizing data or materials, etc.

Of course, in a successful learner's career, schooling should produce all three types of literacy. However, for the unsuccessful or handicapped learner, facility in one or two of these literacies can make a rewarding, satisfying life possible. Too frequently, teachers and parents seem to feel that all three are necessary.

At times teachers and parents must make the conscious decision that limited literacy is an acceptable, even worthwhile, goal. Interestingly, in most cases in which this is true, the learners already know and have agreed to this determination. They know which tasks they can and cannot accomplish. They often recognize their limitations. In counseling children and parents, it often is appropriate to explain these facets of literacy and involve them in the decision.

The skills program is usually not affected by the type of literacy desired but the curriculum is—markedly so. If a youth is dedicated to the mastery of automobile engines and ultimately to their repair, what the individual will read, write, and study is determined by the stratified literacy. However, if literacy is to be the goal, the instructional program may never touch on automobiles. Many learning disabled children are lost because of such decisions made by parents or teachers, while many gifted/learning disabled children are completely maladjusted because stratified literacy is not permitted. Parental counseling is important in this respect.

With nearly all learning disabled children, the first curriculum topics should be stratified if at all possible. Attempts should be made to have the children pursue topics of interest in which they have the best possible background, because past learning is to be employed. This is the most effective situation in which to obtain learning if it is going to happen. It fosters recall and stimulates reinforcing practice. It makes the learning meaningful. At a later date, if general literacy is sought, it can be introduced through the stratified materials.

A youngster engrossed in automobiles can easily become interested in their history, then the accompanying geography and biographies. Trying to force unrelated material into the program causes further negative reactions.

The earlier segments on the language experience approach in Chapter 6, the use of content for instruction (Appendix 6-F), the modified Fernald Procedure (Appendix 6-C), and writing activity (Appendix 6-D) all can be applied to the stratified literacy goal.

Functional literacy should be a part of every instructional program, whether or not the child is handicapped. Children should not die or be injured because they cannot read and understand materials they contact in everyday life. For all learning disabled children, a regular instructional segment should be provided on this type of literacy. Most children, even the gifted or those most disillusioned by school, tend to fit here, usually recognizing the value of such instruction.

One young man who had had a totally unsuccessful experience through nine years of school was discovered to be at the genius level at the end of ninth grade. Academic successes had been few. However, his amazing talent in visualizing machinery and in music led him to organ tuning and repair. His literacy tasks were both stratified and functional. Using the learning techniques described earlier and with a definite set of goals, he learned to read the materials crucial to his future.

Enough general reading ability was developed from these materials to allow him to pass his high school equivalency examination. He never went to college or technical school; they offered him nothing. He was able to become a successful technician, businessman, and parent. One wonders if this would have been so if literacy per se had been the goal demanded of this young man.

Literacy is important, but to many professional families with gifted/learning disabled children it may become too important. Family conflicts, family shame, and child denigration are possible outcomes when the varied possibilities of literacy as a generic term are not explored or are not accepted.

If young children are able to overcome their learning problems, overall literacy can become a goal, but even that might have to be reached through the back door of stratified literacy. The reason for using child interests in instruction is found in this concept.

It appears that the desire for total literacy is uniquely American. Most foreign educational systems very early in a child's career begin fostering stratified literacy concepts. Some children already are being groomed for politics, law, or science early in their lives. Many are not expected to rise to any such levels. This practice carries no stigma to the child but rather opens up a number of new paths. It is almost as if the United States demands that the schools develop "Renaissance" people," highly cultivated and skilled in all or most of the arts and sciences. It would be interesting to discover what the outcome would be for gifted children, especially those with learning disabilities, if they were allowed to pursue their areas of special interest with all their vigor. It is possible that a natural outcome might be true literacy. However, as long as these children are not permitted such a pursuit, the answer never will be known.

Part III

Specific Abilities Unit

Because of the nature of gifted/learning disabled children, certain basic thinking and comprehension abilities should be stressed in their instructional programs. These skills are important to all children, especially those with learning disabilities, but they assume more importance for the gifted.

Specifically, these abilities are:

- word recognition
- classification
- levels of abstraction
- relevancy
- oral language facility
- vocabulary

The thrust of fostering these abilities is to help cope with the vocabulary, flexibility, and adaptability difficulties so often demonstrated by the gifted/learning disabled.

Children from deprived backgrounds can be expected to be gifted; they also can be expected to be learning disabled. However, because of poor language facility, either or both of these factors usually goes unnoticed. For diagnosis to be effective for these children and for those identified as gifted/learning disabled, effective language skills must be developed. Therefore, facility in oral language and vocabulary development also is discussed in this unit, even though it may not be appropriate to most gifted/learning disabled children.

Chapter 7

A Program in Word Recognition

The major system in the reading process called word attack can be viewed as involving two subsystems: word recognition and word analysis or synthesis.

Word analysis or synthesis involves dealing with the elements of words. For gifted/learning disabled children, word analysis might meet their needs better than synthesis. Dealing with wholes is better than dealing with parts. The entire conceptual framework for instruction is predicated on this premise.

The factor to be dealt with first no matter what partial or whole system is being discussed is the importance of word recognition. This subsystem involves dealing with the whole word rather than its parts.

This approach is vital, since in English words get their meaning from their context. A listener or reader produces a noise. The noise becomes a word only when the person is able to give it meaning from the appropriate background of experience and operates in this fashion as a regular procedure.

Frequently, children who have received intensive code-emphasis instruction in reading make very little, if any, use of word recognition skills. In many such programs, children actually are discouraged from bringing to bear as many of their abilities as possible for solving problems with unrecognized words. "Sounding it out" becomes the only acceptable problem-solving technique. Children involved in these programs to any important degree usually are unable to use word recognition clues.

Basically, there are three major elements in word recognition:

1. context clues: the use of meaning
2. language rhythm clues: the use of grammatical and syntactical elements
3. typographical clues: the use of pictures, charts, diagrams, headings, etc.

CONTEXT CLUES

The first and most important of all the word recognition clues is the ability to recognize meaningful and meaningless sentences in oral and written language. Too frequently this elemental aspect of language has not been fostered or may actually have been diminished. To foster this attitude and develop the skill, teachers must insist that language be meaningful. They should:

- Say something meaningless during class or group discussion, noting which children recognize it and which do not; challenge the children to give the meaning; alert them that this will be a regular practice in class.
- Note any meaningless reading during any oral reading but do not correct the child; read the material as the child did and have the pupil evaluate its meaningfulness; encourage the children to note meaninglessness but not as an embarrassment to the reader; be sure the reader has read the material silently before presenting it aloud.
- Insist that children proofread their written work for meaning; try not to point out specific errors; give the children a general impression of where difficulties exist and encourage them to find the problems.

The second component of context clues is the ability to supply meaningful elements into a contextual situation. For example, "We saw a big _____ bear at the zoo." In this sentence the students are looking for a color word or another word that must be appropriate to the meaning. It cannot be yellow or green unless something abnormal has occurred and, once again, the only way this can be ascertained is by using the context.

The third component of context clues is the ability to recognize the influence of the whole context on its specific elements. For example, "We saw a big _____ polar bear at the zoo." It is rather apparent that the addition of "polar" with "at the zoo" provides the reader with a structure that can help determine what the unknown word ought to be.

Once again, the stress always must be on meaning. Gifted/learning disabled children especially need this emphasis. To provide this support, teachers should:

- Omit words during listening activities and have the children supply possible words that might be inserted; ask them, as a group, to evaluate the insertions.
- Provide modified cloze procedures in which the children insert the words they feel appropriate; start with single sentences with one omission, then single sentences with two omissions, and, finally, short paragraphs with multiple missing words, then conduct a group evaluation; be sure to avoid denigrating comments and be willing to spend some time talking over the different

suggestions. (A modified cloze procedure might require all new words the child learned yesterday. Regular cloze is usually based on deleting words by numerical patterns; e.g., every fifth word.)

- Ask the children to substitute synonyms for words in the text during reading instruction.
- Use regular cloze procedure activities for review words and tests.

It is important that success be obtained with these three aspects of context clues before moving into the other areas of word recognition. As noted in Appendix 6-A, for all children, but especially the gifted/learning disabled, it is vital that instruction be organized and consistent and that short-range, attainable goals be developed with the children.

LANGUAGE RHYTHM CLUES

Language rhythm clues are those that arise from the basic patterns of American English. There is a subject-predicate-object relationship for declarative sentences and a different pattern for interrogative sentences. Adjectives are found in certain positions but seldom in others.

These are patterns that children know because if they did not, they could not talk. The words used for these concepts might not be knowns but the concepts are. For example,

Wxe trobld etz vmrbt.

If this meaningless array of letters is viewed as a sentence, the second group looks as if it should be the subject; if it is, the first group is an article, the third is the verb, and the last group is the direct object. This is an example of language rhythm.

Language rhythm might well be subsumed under context but because of a special circumstance it must be dealt with as an entity. The problem in the application of this skill rests with the child's fundamental language pattern. If a pupil is bringing nonstandard English patterns to materials written in standard English, then this type of clue is relatively useless. This may well be one of the major reasons why minority children often go undetected as gifted; even more importantly, it may be so pervasive in evaluations that disabilities are obscured or undetected. The controversy over standard vs. nonstandard English must be resolved before satisfactory application of this concept to word attack can be expected.

Where there is no problem in using standard English, the teacher must continue to place the emphasis on meaning. In doing so, the teacher should:

- present orally a sentence with a grammatical or syntactical error, then ask the children to note it and correct it
- present in writing the same type of sentence and have the children follow the same procedure
- present sentences with blanks and three or four possible words that might be inserted; ask the children to insert the proper words and discuss their reasons; be sure to use grammatical and syntactical variations, e.g., faulty endings, incorrect agreement, etc.
- note areas or lines in writing assignments in which these errors occur and have the children proofread for the mistakes

Because clues provided by context and language rhythm are not available in code emphasis programs, aid for a major learning problem has not been made available to the children affected by the problem of reversals. These problems occur in both reading and writing, yet they often are viewed as the same. The problem in writing is best handled by use of the modified Fernald Procedure, as discussed in Appendix 6-C.

The reading problem is best handled by developing an attitude of reading for meaning and then fostering the use of language rhythm clues. In nearly all reversals, the substituted words are grammatically different. In English, the negative adverb "no" cannot be interchanged with the preposition "on." The past tense of the verb "to be," "was," cannot substitute for "saw," the past tense of the verb "to see."

"My father was the little girl in the tree" is meaningless. Yet many children could read it just that way. It is unfortunate that many remedial reading programs having children with these problems usually deal with the confused words in isolation, where they seldom occur. In context, the reversals might appear but children who are striving for meaning will not accept them and will make the obvious changes. It is astounding the number of children who are aware of this difficulty and yet continue to word-call rather than to think.

For the gifted/learning disabled, this problem appears to be one they could deal with readily because of their better cognitive ability. However, this procedure implies both adaptability and flexibility, which usually is poor in this special group. Many times, these children verbalize what they should do and then, when faced with the problem, become rigid and fail to follow through.

This problem can be dealt with further during a written language activity. Using a modified Fernald Procedure, the teacher asks the child to master one of the confusing pairs. It is not that the pupil does not know "saw" or "was," it is that the youngster does not know one or the other of the two. If one were known, then the confusion would be eliminated. The child can be taught to know whichever is the most important or useful of the confusing pair. Again, the need for integrative instruction for the gifted/learning disabled is apparent. If specific aspects of these children—their innate intelligence, their learning problems, their attitudinal tendencies—are isolated, it is impossible to provide an adequate program. All factors coexist and must be recognized and dealt with as an interacting unit. That unit is the gifted/learning disabled child.

TYPOGRAPHICAL CLUES

Typographical clues are elements of the text that are provided to elucidate, clarify, or structure the material. Their use permits a reader to deal with a word that is not known immediately. In the past these elements either were not mentioned or were listed as picture clues. When picture clues fell into disfavor, after the stress on synthetic phonics developed, the other elements also were disregarded. It is interesting to note that some state competency tests that emphasize functional reading require mastery of these skills, which were frowned upon before the national Right to Read program developed.

Five aspects of this skill are useful in the reading process. They involve the children's ability to:

1. use pictures, graphs, and charts to supplement the text
2. use the text to evaluate pictures, graphs, and charts
3. appreciate the relevancy of pictures, graphs, and charts
4. gain information from pictures, graphs, and charts
5. obtain structure and directions from letters, headings, different print type, etc.

In the area of typographical clues, the first skill listed must be stressed. However the next three can be used as instructional strategies to help with the development of the first. For example, the children read the sentence "The banner was vermilion and gold." The use of the picture can help them understand the words "banner" and "vermilion" if necessary. The meanings can be obtained and the picture then evaluated for correctness.

The children might meet the term "bar graph" and be completely baffled, yet by using the text and having the graph available they can develop an understanding. The multiple meanings of "bar" could be discerned and the important concept of semantic variation enhanced. This technique can help deal with a major vocabulary problem of gifted/learning disabled children—their regimented, limited, narrow vocabulary development.

The fifth skill does not really relate to word recognition. It should be stressed as a comprehension skill. However, with some highly intelligent children the text's organization might bring insight about a word that would not have been learned if the organizing element had not been used.

Ultimately, gifted/learning disabled children must be able to read the vast majority of words at sight. If they must use word analysis skills regularly, then they are using incorrect materials or are operating in an inappropriate fashion. The entire thrust of the word recognition program must be toward the development of sight vocabulary. If youngsters are taught and encouraged to use word recognition techniques, then this goal is more likely to be reached.

Chapter 8

A Program in Classification Skills

Gifted/learning disabled children, as noted earlier, tend to display rigidity, rather than flexibility or adaptability, in their thinking. Therefore, the use of classification activities on a systematic basis can help foster more versatility. Classifying means applying a more abstract term that includes a number of more specific ideas.

The program described here consists of nine steps in the development of the ability to construct outlines. Developing this type of thinking, which is characterized by tight organization, helps many gifted, inflexible children learn to bend. Inherent in its development is the learners' responsibility to perceive samenesses and differences and decide the attributes for selection of items in the outline.

Gifted children with learning difficulties have learned in many cases to mask their problems by not deviating from the steps in a given system. They have found this effective because rigid systems tend to support their inflexibilities. The teacher therefore must be sure that internal procedures in this skills development program never can be performed by using a system. There must be an unpredictable element in every activity.

SYSTEMATIC DEVELOPMENT

This program emphasizes a systematic development of outlining from individual words through paragraph manipulation. It is recommended that at each step no fewer than three but preferably five activities be provided and that there be one activity a day and discussion of its results before material on the next activity is distributed.

Step 1: Grouping Words Into a Given Number of Groups

In this activity the children are given words that can be classified and are told how many groups the teacher wants. For example:

Directions: Put these words into three sensible groups.

cat	chair	shoe
bed	dog	mouse
	sandal	

When the children have finished their groupings, the teacher asks a child to volunteer the groupings. The teacher puts them on the board without comment. Any other child who has different groupings is asked to say them aloud. The teacher then writes them on the board. The teacher asks the two children for the reasons why they used the grouping and involves the others in determining which lists are sensible or whether there are others that are more appropriate. The teacher can accept any groupings that can be justified sensibly.

It is vital as the children prepare their groupings that they write them. This is one more way to develop an organized approach to work and it is helpful in developing a spelling vocabulary.

In preparing activities for the children, the teacher should be sure to use words they know or can find defined in a reference source. It is very beneficial to use words from their experience charts, word banks, or reading matter as the stimuli for these activities. Once again, it is one more way to provide reinforcement.

Step 2: Grouping Words but Determining Number of Groups

In this activity, the children have lost some of the structure provided in step 1. They now must abstract the words and try to find the different aspects that can be generalized. They are forced to see groups of samenesses and recognize that these are the elements that determine the number of groups.

It is at this step that it is useful to introduce the idea of varied levels of abstraction. For example:

Directions: Put these words into sensible groups.

bat	man	ostrich	bass
whale	eagle	pike	penguin

If the teaching procedures listed under step 1 were followed, an interesting situation could arise. One child might provide the following groupings:

bat	eagle	pike
whale	ostrich	bass
man	penguin	

Obviously, these are satisfactory groupings. The child might have decided on mammals, birds, and fish as the classifications even if these labels were not verbalized. However, another child might provide the following different groupings:

bat	whale	man
eagle	penguin	ostrich
	bass	
	pike	

This child might have chosen them by environment, recognizing them as flying, swimming, or walking. Another might suggest that they tended to live in the air, water, and on land. In all three instances if the youngster can state a sensible reason for the grouping, it should be accepted.

For gifted/learning disabled children, this may be the very best procedure to help them learn that there are a number of ways to perceive reality and that it is important to be able to make these adjustments. The problem of inflexibility must be dealt with at every opportunity.

Even though this type of activity is important or even vital, the teacher must be sure that at least one exercise contains no ambiguities, since thinking is desired. Students must not rely on a single system.

Step 3: Grouping Words, Determining Groups, Supplying Titles

In this activity the children must proceed as in the first two steps but must provide a label for each group from their own vocabulary. This opens up the possibility of broadening vocabulary while appreciating levels of abstraction. For example:

Directions: Put these words into three groups and give each group a title.

hat	dog	shirt
socks	cap	tie
	cat	

The activity in step 2 would be useful here with the additional requirement that the children write the titles they have chosen over each group. They should be encouraged to use whatever reference materials they need to accomplish this. The writing in this activity provides further reinforcement. The same give-and-take between and among students should be encouraged as well as frequent rereadings of the lists of words and titles by the teacher and children. The concept that there are a number of ways to look at things should be stressed constantly and practice should be provided.

Step 4: Grouping Specific Words and Classifications

In this activity, the learning in steps 1 and 2 will need to be demonstrated. The children should appreciate that the three capitalized words in the next list make up that which might be called titles. The other problem that many gifted/learning disabled children display is difficulty in recognizing that the title and specifics do not make a group. The following type of activity can be helpful:

Directions: Put these words into sensible groups and give each group a title.

cat	bass	Fish	Mammals
pike	dog	mouse	robin
crow	Birds	eagle	sparrow

The teaching procedure should follow that advocated in steps 1 and 2. The teacher should emphasize that if the students try to classify the different levels of abstraction together, the commonality from idea to idea is missing.

AN INTERLUDE

At this point in the classification program a hiatus can occur. For young children or older students whose problems still are so pronounced that basic study skills are not paramount in the overall program, the successful completion of step 4 could be a satisfactory culmination. For other students whose basic problem is failure to approach their potential, the following four procedures may be of great importance.

Step 5: Grouping Words in Blank Outline with Main Ideas

In this activity children are given an outline with the main ideas supplied. In essence, it is steps 1 and 2 combined with a form supplied as a model. The children are required to take the classifications provided and index the specific items under the appropriate heading. For example:

Directions: Put the words above the outline on the correct lines in the outline.

| chicken | flounder | cow | rockfish |
| pig | duck | trout | turkey |

I. *Birds*
   A. _____
   B. _____
   C. _____

II. *Fish*
   A. _____
   B. _____
   C. _____

III. *Mammals*
   A. _____
   B. _____

In this activity the children have an opportunity to apply the skills developed in steps 1-4.

Step 6: Grouping Words and Classifications in Blank Outline

This step requires the children once again to appreciate the different levels of abstraction of the words provided and to recognize that since the outline has only three classifications, the words must be grouped. For example:

Directions: Fill in the blank outline with the following words.

chicken	flounder	cow	Mammals
pig	duck	trout	rockfish
Birds	turkey	Fish	

I. _____
   A. _____
   B. _____
   C. _____

II. _____
   A. _____
   B. _____
   C. _____

III. _____
   A. _____
   B. _____
   C. _____

When the children usually are successful with steps 5 and 6, another element of organization can be introduced. In the drill work for step 5, the classifications are in alphabetical order. When the children begin the work on step 6, the teacher should encourage them to use this order, then suggest that the subtopics also could be handled that way. It is important to foster thoughtful, organized behavior.

Step 7: Grouping in Blank Outline but Supplying Classification

In this activity the children must abstract and generalize and must produce from their background of experience classifications that not only are appropriate but that also are coordinated.

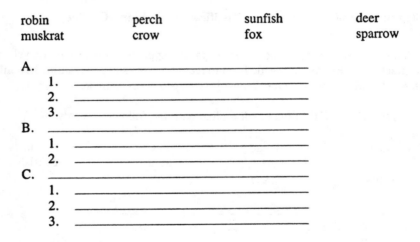

Directions: Fill in the blank outline below with the following words. Supply the words to be used beside the capital letters.

robin   perch   sunfish   deer
muskrat   crow   fox   sparrow

A. _____
   1. _____
   2. _____
   3. _____
B. _____
   1. _____
   2. _____
C. _____
   1. _____
   2. _____
   3. _____

It is interesting to note how many children do not comprehend that there are only two items under B. The teacher must not caution them about such things but should let them have to live with impetuous lack of thinking. The teacher also should try to ascertain whether there was any order in the subtopics.

For steps 5, 6, and 7, the same basic procedures are followed as those suggested earlier. The teacher should have the outlines on the board, and ask the children to discuss and evaluate each other's suggestions in a positive fashion. It is important to note which children are struggling and provide them with more than the normal opportunities. Since these activities should be done independently, there is no reason for a child who requires it not to receive extra help.

Step 8: Outlining a Paragraph

It is at this point that the direct application of the abilities begins. It is here that the children need to recognize that there are certain elements in the paragraph that are coordinated and therefore can be classified and that in most cases they will have to provide these classifications from their vocabularies.

The first paragraph to be outlined should be one that is developed from the last outline of step 7. For example:

> The small swamp near our house was my favorite place to see animals. On the banks of the swamp, you could find the prints of a deer, a fox, or a small muskrat. In the water you could see sunfish and perch. In the tall grasses you could see robins, sparrows, and crows. I loved to go there.

There are a number of different ways to outline that paragraph correctly. However, once it has been done, it is helpful to show the children the outline from which it was prepared. It also is interesting to note how many children recognize the paragraph as the outline already used in step 7.

This step can and should be reinforced by using content materials of various types. Multiple paragraphs should be introduced once success with single paragraphs is a regular occurrence. However, the teacher should be sure not to introduce fictional materials into the procedures. They are not meant to be outlined and generally offer no basic value in developing this ability.

A SECOND INTERLUDE

Once again, a point of culmination has been reached. For students who need this basic ability as a study skill, the program can be halted. However, for many of the gifted/learning disabled this process should be used to promote written expression. Many very bright children should be encouraged to do more than "creative writing." Help and guidance in technical writing should be a part of their program where it is appropriate. Procedures, specifications, and detailed explanations are included. There is no pretense that this classification program will develop technical writing but it may well be a good first step; for some children it has opened up a world of writing they never knew was available to them.

Because of the vocabulary problems of gifted/learning disabled children and their tendency to have specific areas of interest, regular written language programs in school often have been unresponsive to their needs. For children whose interests are geared to content area subject matter, step 9 can be a rewarding activity.

Step 9: Developing a Simple Paragraph from an Outline

In this activity the teacher presents an outline of material and asks the children to write a paragraph from it. In essence, it is the introduction to good technical writing. The preparation of an outline always is a useful step before attempting to construct a paragraph. For example:

Swamp Animals I Loved to Watch

Directions: Use the following outline to write a paragraph that contains this information.

A. Birds
    1. crow
    2. robin
    3. sparrow
B. Fish
    1. perch
    2. sunfish
C. Mammals
    1. deer
    2. fox
    3. muskrat

Once again it can be useful to take the last activity in step 8 and convert it for use at step 9. It must be understood that step 9 cannot really be developed unless some basic research skills have been or are being formed at the same time.

Throughout this suggested plan of action it has been noted that a positive interaction be maintained between students and teacher, and students and students. The teacher should keep the material at the pupils' self-evaluation level and not try to become involved with grading. Teacher evaluation also should focus on the diagnostic aspects revealed by careful observation of the behaviors.

The children should not be rushed through the sequence. A week or more spent on each step can be most productive; however, with certain gifted/learning disabled children, their inherent rigidity may make it necessary to stay on a given step for a much longer time.

VARIATIONS

There are other forms for presenting material to provide children with the opportunity to use classification skills. For example:

Directions: Read the sentences below and cross out the one word that does not fit the classification.

Pear, apple, radish, and peach are all fruits.
Toe, finger, arch, and heel are all foot parts.

In the above activity the children must use the classification and then determine which of the items does not fit it.

Directions: Fill in the blank so that the sentence makes sense.

Pear, apple, and peach are all _____.
Toe, heel, and arch are all _____.

In this format the children must classify the items. It is the same thinking process as used with a column.

Directions: Cross out the word in each line that does not belong.

Pear, apple, radish, peach
Finger, toe, heel, arch

This activity requires a generalization before the correct response can be made. The teacher also can use the above format but require in the directions that the children state why they eliminated the one word.

In an activity requiring justification, the teacher should be sure to ascertain the type of reasoning and determine whether it is based on classification or on concept development. For example:

Directions: Pick the word in each line that does not belong and state why.

Alps   Andorra   Rocky   Andes

There are two correct answers. One response might be Rocky, the other Andorra. The justifications are the major concern. One response might be Rocky because it begins with R. This is not a satisfactory response. With that type of reasoning, an answer could be Alps because it starts with Al, which precedes either of the two An words.

The response sought is Andorra because the others are mountains and it is a principality. Even the answer Rocky is acceptable if the justification is that all the other words begin with A. Of course, anyone teaching social studies might be disheartened by that correct response.

Directions: Fill in the blanks with the appropriate item.

Apple, pear, and _____ are all fruits.
Heel, arch, and _____ are all foot parts.

In this activity the children must index. They must go back into their repertoire of concepts and specifics and find the appropriate word to make the sentence sensible.

All of these formats can be used as teaching, reinforcing, or application techniques wherever they seem appropriate in the basic nine-step sequence.

Chapter 9

A Program in Levels of Abstraction

Words in English are different both quantitatively and qualitatively. The quantitative differences are in the spelling, or letter sequences. The qualitative differences exist in the amount of information a given word in a given content conveys.

For many gifted/learning disabled children, the problems with flexibility and adaptability noted so often in this text are operative in this area, too. The major area of influence, however, seems to be vocabulary extension. This lack of appreciation of varying amounts of data within a word and its context leads to stilted usage and limited expression.

A program to remediate this problem should begin by sensitizing the children to the abstracting process; that is, they must be able to appreciate the parts of the whole. In some youngsters the gestalt—the whole concept—is so powerful that the parts seem to be obscured. These children usually demonstrate severe difficulty in developing, maintaining, and using word analysis or synthesis skills. Rules for attacking words are useless if the individual cannot perceive the elements of the words that must be used. Many gifted/learning disabled children demonstrate this problem to a less debilitating degree but it is apparent if an examiner is sensitive to it.

The following sequences of learning experiences have been helpful in this respect for all children. However, teachers should be aware that this type of procedure for the learning disabled might generate some initial negative responses. Many of these children find this type of demand by teachers very vexing.

In conducting a program to develop an appreciation of the levels of abstraction in gifted/learning disabled children, the teacher should:

- Start with a common animal, such as a dog, and have the children provide the attributes that generally lead to the concept of a dog. Then do the same for a cat. Note the attributes as the children provide them. Then use another vertebrate, such as a bird, and follow the same procedure. The material on the chalkboard might be as follows:

dog	*cat*	*bird*
four legs	fur	two legs
two ears	four legs	two wings
tail	tail	tail
hair	two ears	feathers
claws	two eyes	two eyes
eats	eats	sings
	claws	eats

- Have the children note that if the dog and cat headings were reversed, the words still would be right. Try to develop with them the fact that because they have not abstracted enough details, the classification could be either animal or mammal. Get the children to note that adding the appropriate vocal sound and retractable (cat) or nonretractable (dog) claws permits the differentiation. Have them note that in the bird column if certain attributes are used, the three can be put together as animals but the addition of feathers and wings makes it possible to split the groups into mammals and birds.
- Have the students note that the common attributes are used to put the two realities together (formation of a concept); the uncommon things separate them (differentiation of concepts).
- Point out that all three animals eat, fur makes dog and cat (mammals) different from bird, and noise differences and retractable claws separate cat from dog.

Once regular success has been demonstrated with these understandings, more demanding types of activities can be employed. The teacher then should:

- Provide two sentences about some experiences using different levels of abstraction. Have students note the differences in degree of meaning. For example:

  The car killed an animal.
  The car killed a squirrel.

- Provide three or four terms from common experiences and have the students list them in degree of information. For example:

Directions: Read a column of words below. Then rearrange the column so that the first word provides the least information and the bottom word the most.

mammal	mountain	fossil fuel
dog	geographical feature	fuel
animal	Himalayan mountain	coal
living thing	Mt. Everest	

- When the children report their listings, accept the list whether right or wrong, and discuss the material. Have them practice their abstracting skills in the group. Make sure the items are so precise that a correct, unambiguous response is possible.
- Have children use a text and insert higher level or lower level abstractions into sentences, then discuss the meaning changes.

This technique is especially important with content materials. The children should note how higher levels of abstractions in sciences can make communication less clear, as noted with the animal and squirrel example above. It also is important to have them note how much faster communication can be through the use of higher level terms, but only if the appropriate abstracted information is available to the reader or listener. Listening, speaking, reading, and writing should be incorporated whenever possible. The term *level of abstraction* can be developed as a vocabulary item with the children. However, many children might prefer to say *tells more* or *tells less*.

If a need exists in this area of learning, this material should be incorporated on a regular basis. The teacher should not indulge in an incidental exposure of these procedures to the children. If this ability is worth learning, it is worthy of consistent instruction. It can be readily integrated into nearly all language activities. Work in classification both supports and requires an understanding of varied levels of abstraction.

Chapter 10

A Program in Appreciating Relevancy

Relevance is the quality of being pertinent to, or properly applying to, the case in hand. In other words, things fit or go together. This perception often is poorly developed in gifted/learning disabled children. In their rigidity, the appreciation that one behavior could be pertinent to a number of situations is often disturbing. Therefore, it is important that activities be provided to foster the appreciation and acceptance of relevancy.

Initially, the teacher should use a common behavior and have the children try to state as many situations as possible in which it could be relevant—for example, washing their hands. This activity could be relevant to cleaning up:

- before dinner
- after playing
- after working in a garden
- after going to the bathroom

The list could be augmented by a number of other situations, of course. It is important for the teacher to write the responses and have the children read them repeatedly. This, once again, is excellent reinforcement.

A response should be accepted even if its relevancy is not apparent; the teacher then should question the pupil as to why it should be considered relevant. In many cases, special circumstances in a child's life may make an answer quite relevant. This type of oral activity at the group level should continue until the students are comfortable with it and make rather quick responses.

In the next stage, an activity is presented and the children must provide relevant behaviors. For example, getting ready to eat. The relevant behaviors might be:

- washing the hands
- setting the table

- placing the chairs
- calling the other children to the table

Once again the suggested procedures for the first stage should be followed so that discussion are rereading are carried on as a natural part of the classroom activity.

When the children have demonstrated in the group that they can perform these thinking tasks, independent activities should be introduced. A good way to accomplish this is to provide each child with a work sheet to be filled in as part of the follow-up activity or homework. If the material is sent home, the result may not be what is desired. Parents of gifted/learning disabled children may be reluctant to permit an error, even if it is important information for the teacher. Parents' coaching and, in some cases, actual performing of the work is not uncommon. It generally is better to have the children do all of this type of work in school.

Follow-up activity is useful as practice and application of relevancy. For example:

Directions: Below on the left are four activities. To the right are nine related things you might do. Put the number of the behavior beside any of the activities where it might occur. Activities may have more than one number beside them.

_____ attending a square dance	1. get wet
	2. hold hands with a stranger
_____ cleaning the basement	3. wear nice clothes
	4. wear a warm coat
_____ going to church	5. eat
	6. laugh a lot
_____ building a snowman	7. listen to music
	8. use tools
	9. walk or use a car

When the children have finished the activity, the teacher should discuss it with them as a group, preferably in the next class meeting. It is important to note whether they can maintain their reasoning for the relevant choices. With this special population, the one-day (or more) delay often is necessary since some of these children cannot maintain a flexible, adaptive attitude after a night at home. This inflexibility can be reinforced or demanded by the home; as a result, daily perceived gains often are quite transitory. If such is the case, discussions with the parents are absolutely necessary.

Similar activities are easy to devise. They should include current vocabulary, present and past conceptual areas, and items of individual interest. They can center on personal behavior, social adjustment, personal hygiene, the curriculum, and any other topic appropriate to the group or individual.

It is important to reiterate that group discussion to promote individual understanding is absolutely necessary. Left to their own egocentric views, the pupils might never achieve this very necessary change of perception.

Chapter 11

A Program for Oral Language Facility

When children learn to express themselves thoughtfully and without fear, when they learn to listen and to take an interest in what others have to say, they have developed a skill that probably correlates with success in life more than anything else taught in school. (Glasser, 1969)

When working with many disadvantaged children either in the city or the rural areas, two factors in language development become obvious:

1. These children have pronounced difficulty communicating with people other than those in their very close environment.
2. It is extremely difficult for people to communicate with them.

These two difficulties are intertwined, yet separate. Certain factors bring this paradox about.

LANGUAGE, LABELING, COMMUNICATION

Children in language-disadvantaged environments have little understanding of the true function of language. In many of their homes, language is used to manipulate them rather than to communicate ideas to them. (This may well be a solid definition of a language-disadvantaged environment.) A parent says, "Be quiet," or "Get out of here." The idea is to move the child in some way. In many homes with no language disadvantage, the same movements are necessary to run a household. However, the language is slightly different. The parent may say, "Be quiet, *I want to listen to the radio*," or "Get out of here, *I want to run the vacuum cleaner*."

Another problem is a general lack of labeling of things and ideas in language disadvantaged homes. Once again the movement of children rather than communication or language development is the parents' goal. They are inclined to say, "Put that away," rather than "Put the milk in the refrigerator." Again, both the interrelationship of those two factors and their uniqueness are pointed up.

In a school where an attempt was being made to facilitate overall language development, the program was stymied because basic communication was hindered seriously. Without communication there can be no teaching. In a procedure involving household words and things, the children did not recognize and, therefore, could not use sensibly the term "sink," meaning the kitchen sink. However, they knew how to use the sink. In another school, students called the small alarm clock on the teacher's desk a "wake-up bell." In both situations the correct label was not in their listening or speaking vocabulary.

The goal of this program is to provide material and procedures to be used to meet the oral language and communication needs of language-disadvantaged children. It is not to be considered a reading readiness program. Rather, it is designed to facilitate communication so that teaching in general can be accomplished. The major thrust is to have the pupils develop a listening vocabulary, because without one, teaching is impossible and a reading vocabulary becomes merely making noises.

Too frequently, this type of program is conceived as being suitable only for very poor children but many children from more affluent homes are just as handicapped in this respect as the poor. In some cases, the program might be considered too elemental for older students. However, if progress is to be made in helping these children, any changes are merely in substance, not form. The same tasks have to be carried out. It is hoped that through this program educators can discover a number of previously unidentified gifted children; possibly those whose development has been stymied by learning disabilities can be provided with appropriate help.

BASIC PROCEDURES

The basic concept in this program is to provide the children who need it with some basic experience that can be labeled and discussed. The discussion is directed toward recognizing the need for communication and fostering basic listening skills.

In this program the teacher has four major objectives:

1. to provide interesting and commonly shared experiences
2. to initiate dialogue about the experiences
3. to encourage discussion between and among the children
4. to prepare preprogram and postprogram evaluations

Providing Experiences

A number of specific areas (listed later) might be included other than those described here. The program should begin with small group instruction, preferably 10 to 12 children in kindergarten to second grade. It requires the use of manipulative objectives. For this discussion, small zoo animal figures are used since most cities have a zoo where the real animal can be observed. To avoid overstimulating the children, only two or three animal models should be provided. If possible, two of them should not be highly stimulating but one should be exotic: a lion, a tiger, and a giraffe. Because of its exotic features, the giraffe lends itself to vocabulary development.

The teacher should start by asking the children to name the animals. If they cannot do so, the teacher should. It is important that the children recognize the names of the animals and respond correctly when a name is used. When the teacher says, "Pick up the lion," it is vital that they do this as a first step. It is not initially important that the children use the words. The listening vocabulary must be firmly fixed before the speaking vocabulary can be developed.

Once the children have labeled the animals, the teacher can begin to develop the attributes of each one. However, it might be better to stress the giraffe because it offers a variety of ideas:

- tall (it is the tallest of all animals)
- spotted (model must be correctly spotted)
- long-legged
- horned (the teacher should point out the protuberances even though they are not true horns)

When the children have assimilated this information, a trip to the local zoo is appropriate. However, it should not be an all-day or a general visit; rather it should be a specific visit to see the giraffe and get information about it. This should include how the giraffe drinks, what and how it eats, how it sleeps, etc.

Back in the classroom the children should be given an opportunity to talk about the giraffe, not the trip. It is important to direct the discussion toward the precise experience that was set up in the classroom, rather than the general trip experience, that each pupil could structure individually.

The discussion should attempt to bring out the facts learned at the zoo about the animal investigated. Appropriate pictures could be used to stimulate or revitalize ideas. The teacher should observe the children as they begin to use the appropriate speaking vocabulary. If possible, activities should be planned in which the children who are using the language become involved in team activities such as:

- having a speaking child suggest to a listening child the coloring of certain parts in an animal drawing
- having all the children do an animal jigsaw puzzle together, with a speaking child calling the names of the parts
- having the children play a concentration game with two or three pairs of animal cards; they should be required to use the animal names before a pair can be accepted

Initiating Dialogue

Before going to the zoo, the children should understand the concept of a zoo. If possible, the teacher should bring in pictures and discuss the relevant concept of the zoo: a safe, restricted, pleasant place to look at animals from many parts of the world, not just from the local area. Group discussions can bring out reasons for visiting the zoo but these should be kept pertinent to the specific animal under discussion. Three or four ideas should be established for which answers are to be sought at the zoo. Finally, each child should pick out one of those questions to take to the zoo and seek the answer. Some questions might be:

- What do the animals eat and how are they fed?
- How do they drink water?
- How and where do they sleep?
- What are the colors and what kinds of markings do they have? (Children will need to understand color recognition words for this.)
- How tall is an adult animal and how tall is a young one or a baby?

This procedure is vital if the program is to succeed. For many children it will provide real reasons for recalling questions, looking for answers, and framing verbal replies. It is of utmost importance that each child be able to verbalize the reason for going to the zoo and the teacher must be sure the verbalization really makes sense. The teacher should have a list with each child's name and question. Before the trip, the teacher should spot check to determine whether the pupils are remembering their purposes and questions.

At the zoo, the children should be allowed a general view of the plant and then should proceed to the giraffe cage. While they are looking, the teacher should circulate among them and refresh their memories about their specific goals there. If a guide talks with the group, the teacher should ask that the ideas in which the pupils are interested be covered. When a point is made, it should be called to the attention of the children who could use the information. The teacher should try to have the class leave the zoo as quickly as possible through areas that are not highly stimulating. Fresh, stimulating experiences with other animals might obliterate the ideas being worked on.

Discussion of the giraffe should begin as soon as possible—on the bus or once the children are back in the classroom. No other topic except the giraffe should be discussed at this time. The following type of approach can be tried:

Teacher:	What place did you visit today?
Response:	Zoo
Teacher:	Billy, what animal did we go there to visit?
Response:	Giraffe
Teacher:	Billy, what did you want to find out about the giraffe?
Response:	(Billy replies with his question.)
Teacher:	Mary, what was Billy trying to find out?
Response:	(Should be same as Billy's.)
Teacher:	1. (If Mary responds incorrectly) Billy, will you tell us again, repeat your question? (Note here the use of *repeat* in the immediate context and *question* for trying to find out.)
	2. (If Mary responds correctly or after she responds correctly) Billy, what answer did you get to your question?
Response:	(Billy answers)
Teacher:	Who else had the same question as Billy? Did you get the same answer? Tell us what your answer is. Mary, you heard the answers. Do you think they are right? If I asked you their question, what would your answer be?

This type of continuous back-and-forth dialogue, teacher to individual, child to child, and teacher to group, should be continued until obvious signs of waning interest indicate it should be terminated. It is important at this point in the initial discussion that each child should have been given a chance to discuss the questions and answers and to participate in the analysis of other pupils' questions and answers.

While this is going on, the teacher should be making notes about each child's response and have the material available for quick reference when the discussion is started again. The teacher also should be prepared with activities of various kinds to reinforce ideas. Drawing and coloring activities are appropriate, as well as those noted earlier.

On the following day, a group activity should be developed. The stimulation might start through the use of pictures. Once begun, the teacher should use notes to refresh the children's memories about what they had said. It is at this time that higher level vocabulary can be placed in juxtaposition to the child's ready vocabulary so as to broaden the overall listening vocabulary.

For example, the teacher might initially say, "What did we ride on to get to the zoo?" As the familiarity with the concept grows, it can be phrased, "What vehicle did we ride on to get to the zoo?" If the children do not respond, the teacher should press them to identify and understand the concept involved: "How did we get there? We got there on a bus. I asked you, What vehicle did we ride on to get to the zoo? What word does vehicle mean?" The children should be pushed until they say "bus" and "vehicle." This is followed with further developmental questions such as:

What vehicle does Santa Claus ride in?
What vehicle do I ride in to get to school?
What vehicle do the children ride around the street?

The teacher should try first to have the children recognize the word but not to use it immediately. The teacher should go through a magazine or a stack of pictures and ask the children to raise their hands when they see a vehicle. This is the basis for the whole program: the development of a strong listening vocabulary.

Encouraging Discussion

In promoting language usage and verbalization in the language-disadvantaged, it is necessary to deal with these children in small groups. Having three or four children involved in a discussion permits each one to have a role but does not let the amount of material verbalized to accumulate to such a degree that the pupils lose the point or become overwhelmed. It means that for some time, the teacher will have to be involved to provide some basic direction. However, the adult presence should not inhibit language usage. It is important that the children be given the opportunity to talk when they feel they have something to say.

The use of anecdotal notes discussed in Appendix 6-E is helpful if the discussion begins to wane. The teacher might say, "Billy, you said you liked the lion best of all. Now that we have looked at the giraffe, do you still like the lion best?" An answer can be countered with an appropriate "Why?" or "Why not?"

The teacher should try to provide team games (two students) or activities where communication is required. Cooperative paintings on which each pupil has a panel can elicit conversation if team or group planning is required.

At this time, elaboration of the trip can begin or plans for the next experience and trip prepared. In elaborating on the trip, the children might want to build a small zoo out of cardboard and make individual cages for specific animals. During these activities, the teacher should begin to introduce specific useful vocabulary: admission, gate, guide, moat, bars, pen (animal pen), keeper, veterinarian, etc.

In planning for the next trip, an evaluation must be made. Are the children now ready in terms of concentration and amount of self-direction to approach the task as two, or possibly three, teams? This decision is the teacher's. If they are going to work in teams, then the teams should grow out of shared interest. However, limits are necessary at this time—the children cannot be given complete freedom. The teacher should introduce two or three animals to be investigated and permit each child to choose the group in which to work.

The teacher should try to get each group to recall what was done for the first trip and what should be prepared for this one. When each group completes its planning, the teacher should call them all together and have each unit tell the others what animal it is interested in and what goals have been set. The other group members should be encouraged to comment on the information supplied. Meaningful remarks about another group's concern should be noted. Children who were not able to offer information for another group probably will need a continuation of this program until their overall communication skills develop and their general social maturity increases.

Preparing Evaluations

The most difficult part of this project is evaluation. No really reliable objective measures of skill development are being tried here.

Of more importance, in any case, are the subjective evaluations of the teachers and other staff members. It is important that persons not intimately connected with the program make the initial subjective evaluation on each child; when the program is concluded, these same individuals should conduct reevaluations and compare the initial and final observations.

If a diagnostician has performed the initial evaluation, the analysis should have involved some diagnostic observation. For the evaluation process, this same procedure should be carried out. It is important that direct comparisons are made among initial and subsequent behaviors.

It also is beneficial to give both the program and nonprogram children an initial evaluation battery and a final battery and then perform the necessary statistical evaluations to obtain some objective measures and interpretations. A primary mental abilities test could be of some value. However, it must be remembered that all tests are to some degree language bound and the results must be interpreted as reflecting present, not potential, functioning. This one lack of understanding has kept many gifted/learning disabled children from being recognized as gifted.

Finally, a detailed evaluation of the children should be carried out at the end of the year. Progress of a control group should be compared against the progress of the program group. Various areas should be evaluated, especially those of language development that can be measured.

SPECIFIC TECHNIQUES FOR SPECIFIC SKILLS

Abstracting

This involves helping children see the parts of the whole (see Chapter 9 on abstracting). The teacher should:

- Use concrete objects around the classroom, such as a chair or table, and help children give the specific parts (being sure to use only one object at a time initially). Write name of item; under name, list parts. Drawings may be placed alongside the words as an aid. For example:

Chair

legs or four legs
back
seat
rungs (taught if not known)

- Do the same thing with a table or a desk, e.g.:

Table

legs or four legs
top

- Use the same procedures with farm animals, zoo animals, vehicles, etc. Be sure that the two or three items used have common attributes.

Generalizing

This involves helping children see the common aspects of objects and ideas (see Chapter 8 on classification). The teacher should:

- Use the listings made—the real objects if necessary—and have children note the common elements; e.g., chairs and tables have legs but this is their only common attribute.
- Have children look around the room or use pictures to find things that have common qualities. Note the children who cling to stereotyped responses and those who begin to apply the principle to objects and ideas not discussed in class.

- Begin to do this on a purely verbal level with children who demonstrate a grasp of the concept. "How are a dog and a horse the same?" Encourage precise vocabulary for attributes selected. Comparisons could include house-school, bike-car, kitchen-classroom, socks-shirt, Mary-Ellen, Mary-Bill, etc.

Labeling

This involves helping children learn to attach correct labels to experiences. The teacher should:

- Teach children correct labels for classroom facilities. Label those that can be identified with handwritten tags. Note that labeling with tags works best when children need the tags to identify items. A tag on the door carries little significance since most children do not need such a label to handle the required behavior. A tag on the crayon box, however, can be useful if pupils need crayons. If the crayon box is kept in one place, then its tag, like the door's, is unnecessary. Move whatever can be moved, to demonstrate the value of knowing labels. Children will need to know the terms to find what they need.
- Try to use a consistent label until all the children have it firmly in their listening vocabulary. From that time on, begin to use some appositives to broaden the vocabulary as well as extend it.
- Have the children begin to use descriptive adjectives with the correct labels, e.g., "Yes, this is a truck and that is a bus. What else can you tell me about them? Good! It is a green truck and a yellow bus."
- Have children collect or sort pictures that are included under a label; e.g., cut out any pictures that show a car or vehicle or put all the pictures of cars in a certain pile.

Appreciating Levels of Abstraction

This involves helping children appreciate qualitative differences in words (again see Chapter 9 on abstraction). The teacher should:

- Have children select a list of concrete objects that obviously are related (chair, table, desk), then present them with the more abstract term, furniture, if they cannot provide it themselves. If the term is new, be sure to treat it exactly as was suggested earlier in this chapter. Listening skills must be the first and foremost objective of the program.

- Present children with objects, pictures, or words, if appropriate, that have been grouped. Encourage them to pick one of three choices that encompass the grouped material—e.g., show chairs, tables, and desks and ask them to pick games, toys, or furniture.
- Use same types of materials as in the preceding paragraph but put all the items together. Help children find the three items that go together in the classification. In this area, do not attempt to move too fast; take enough time on each step to ensure good control of the material.
- Use the same procedures as above but increase the levels of abstraction or vary the term, e.g., instead of cats, dogs, fish, use animals and pets; instead of water and soda use drinks and beverages; instead of shoes, socks, and sneakers, use footwear and apparel.
- Provide a list of words that describes one thing and have children decide which word gives the most information, least information, etc., or list the items in ascending or descending order; e.g., animal, dog, Lassie, living thing can become living thing, animal, dog, Lassie.

Defining Words

If the program developed in these materials is successful, the children involved in it should begin to be able to handle oral language with greater facility. However, to make this possible, direct guidance in defining words can be helpful.

There are many ways to structure definitions, synonyms, apposition, etc. However, because of the nature of this program, a way to define words is suggested as a starting point. Once reasonable facility is attained with this procedure, others can be introduced.

This is a very important aspect of this program for gifted/learning disabled children. With their problems in flexibility and adaptability, providing a structure is important initially. The security this structure provides can prevent emotional reactions. When a new format for definition is introduced, it must be done slowly and with an indication of how it fits with the one already suggested.

The procedure is based on the use of the stimulus word as the subject of the definition, the verb "to be" as the predicate, and a classification or specific item as the predicate nominative. The predicate nominative is elaborated on when necessary. The teacher should:

- Have children select (or give them) a stimulus word and have them say what it is with a minimal number of words, e.g., chair. A chair is furniture or a piece of furniture. Do not accept "something to sit on"; a table can be sat upon.
- Have children elaborate on the predicate nominative, e.g., "A chair is a piece of furniture usually made of wood that is meant to sit on, and a table is a

piece of furniture usually made of wood that is used to hold objects such as dishes." The children should be rather well versed in levels of abstraction before they can define words well. Be sure they have opportunities to use words that are either more abstract or less abstract as predicate nominatives.

- Have children define both dog and animal, or chair and furniture. Encourage them to evaluate the meaningfulness of the definitions.
- Present true definitions that are more or less meaningful and ask the children to decide which part of the definition helps or hinders them. For example, "An eland is a mammal," then, "An eland is a kind of antelope with two spiral twisted horns."
- Encourage children to use meaningful definitions whenever the possibility arises.

OTHER STIMULI FOR DEVELOPING LANGUAGE

If the use of zoo animals and the zoo is impractical, other areas can be used to provide stimulation. Some of them might require variations of the procedures outlined for the zoo animals but the basic approach remains the same.

I. Stimuli in the School
   A. Physical factors
      1. drinking fountains
      2. fire doors
      3. stairs and stairwells
      4. bulletin boards
      5. kitchen appliances

   B. Geographic factors
      1. offices
      2. halls
      3. cafeteria
      4. entrances and exits
      5. play areas
      6. boiler room

II. Stimuli in the Classroom
   A. Physical factors
      1. closets
      2. sinks
      3. lavatories with fixtures
      4. lighting with switches
      5. types and operation of windows
      6. heating equipment

    B. Geographical features
      1. front and back of room
      2. independent area
      3. teaching area
      4. follow-up area

    C. Activities
      1. cooking
      2. animal care and observation
      3. plant growing
      4. art work

III. Stimuli in the Community
    A. Stores: food, clothing, hardware, etc.
    B. Fire station
    C. Police station
    D. Service station
    E. Manufacturing plants
    F. Ships and waterfront facilities
    G. Bridges and ferries
    H. Botanical gardens
    I. Arboretum
    J. Museums
    K. Historical sights
    L. Veterinarian's office and kennels
    M. Pet shops
    N. Water treatment facilities
    O. Water bodies: river, brook, lake, pond, etc.
    P. Roads and street safety (especially sign recognition)
    Q. Governmental facilities: post office, navy yard, airfield, etc.
    R. Transportation facilities: trolley, bus, train, etc., and where they are housed and repaired
    S. Buildings and their facilities: foyers, canopies, elevators, escalators, etc.

Some aspects of the oral language facility program have value for nearly all gifted/learning disabled children. Individual teachers must decide that in respect to individual pupils. However, in any resource room where this suggested program is tried, a conscious effort must be made to identify children who suddenly blossom because of the structured approach and their recognition of fundamental developmental processes (Barbe & Renzulli, 1975; Karnes & Collins, 1978; Marland, 1972). Although 3 to 5 percent of all children are possibly gifted, a number of educators of the gifted have postulated that 50 to 80 percent of these will be unidentified. It seems apparent that identification might be improved by observing them as they react and develop in planned programs. For the gifted/learning disabled child, this type of procedure, unfortunately, might be an only chance.

REFERENCES

Barbe, W.B., & Renzulli, J.S. *Psychology and education of the gifted*. New York: Irvington Publishers, 1975, p. 23.

Glasser, W. *Schools without failure*. New York: Harper & Row, Publishers, Inc., 1969.

Karnes, F.A., & Collins, E.C. State definitions on the gifted and talented: A report and analysis. *Journal for the Education of the Gifted*, 1978.

Marland, S.P. *Education of the gifted and talented*. Report to the Congress of the United States by the U.S. Commissioner of Education. Washington, D.C.: U.S. Government Printing Office, 1972.

Chapter 12

A Program for Vocabulary Development

Vocabulary development is something that is stressed at all levels in all schools. Most teachers consider it one of their most difficult tasks. Yet, school systems seldom enunciate a philosophy and a psychology of vocabulary development.

THE BASIC ELEMENTS

It must be remembered that vocabulary is a generic or umbrella term. It encompasses many different language facets:

- There is simple language acquisition, which is really the assembling of vocabulary items. This often is looked on as the height of the vocabulary.
- There is the expansion of vocabulary, the use of more precise words based on the appreciation of the context. This is in effect the breadth of vocabulary.
- There is the understanding of nuances, sarcasm, emphasis, etc., as the individual moves into greater sophistication.
- There is the stratified vocabulary, words indigenous to a specialty field of any kind, jargon, etc.

All four of these facets still fall under vocabulary as a term and must be so recognized in instructional programs.

In a program designed to meet the needs of gifted/learning disabled children, the acquisition aspect of vocabulary development has an important place. It does not appear to be a major element in the life of children identified as gifted. They usually do well on straight vocabulary measures. However, the unidentified gifted child is another case. There are two types of these pupils who must be recognized: (1) the child whose learning problem is in language acquisition and (2) the socioeconomically deprived child whose life style does not foster language development. Both of these types need a language acquisition program primarily for diagnostic reasons. (A program appropriate to these children is detailed in Chapter 11, on developing oral language facility. The diagnostic/prescriptive aspects are discussed in Chapter 5 on the socioeconomically deprived child.)

The second aspect of vocabulary development—broadening—is of particular importance to most gifted/learning disabled children. As has been mentioned, they tend to acquire vocabulary in depth but not with semantic variation. Their vocabularies tend to be almost stereotypical. A basic approach to this problem must be through emphasis on context. These children must recognize that in most cases a number of terms can be used for a concept and that these are determined by the contextual setting. (For a detailed discussion of a procedure to accomplish this, see Chapter 7 on word recognition.)

The more sophisticated aspects of nuances, sarcasm, etc., are developed after the pupils become skillful in the use of context. Learning disabled children as a group tend to be very literal. A word means what it means. This is why a teacher of the learning disabled seldom can succeed in classroom or individual control by using sarcasm or innuendo. After one rather serious transgression, a teacher declared sarcastically, "You are really very helpful"—and the child beamed with pleasure. The sarcasm was full and rich. The child smiled but was confused because he knew he had done wrong, yet the literal words were "very helpful."

It is important to note that much time can be wasted in this area. Some of these children may never resolve this problem and an overly intense program may only bring on control problems that are not necessary. A program should, of course, be tried and, if unsuccessful, attempted again later. But at some point, the reality that these children never will really be successful in this area must be accepted.

On the other hand, most gifted/learning disabled children do well in stratified vocabulary. This is especially true in areas of intense interest. For many, sophistication of language in very specific areas is a characteristic. This is evidenced not only in vocabulary but also in overall language facility. A child might be an expert on dinosaurs yet be unable to relate a fable or fairy tale or discuss any components. Once again, a sound program might very well focus on the child's strengths, develop them, and use them to attempt an overall broadening educational effort. It also must be recognized that such an approach might not be successful.

DEVELOPMENTAL TECHNIQUES

There are a number of specific techniques that should be included in any vocabulary development program, such as (1) context, (2) synonyms and antonyms, and (3) roots—English and foreign.

Teachers and children alike are told that the best way to expand their vocabulary is through wide reading. This probably is true under certain conditions.

- The individual must use context clues reasonably well if wide reading is to help with vocabulary development. If this is not true, then wide reading might do little.
- Wide reading might extend the depth of vocabulary but not the breadth. Readers get primarily whatever meaning is in the text.
- The most troublesome aspect of this statement is that individuals must read to improve vocabulary. Many learning disabled children, even gifted ones, do not enjoy reading and for many it is or has been a painful process. Reading may never become something for them to use in leisure time. If gifted/learning disabled children do such reading, it tends to be in their interest areas, in which they already have a more than adequate vocabulary.

The implications of these ideas are that deliberate techniques should be used in the children's programs to foster vocabulary development. The use of word recognition skills was mentioned earlier. That concept highlights an important philosophic understanding: printed words do not mean anything in themselves. In English, printed words represent sounds; they are not ideograms. In and of themselves, words cannot give meaning. The listener or reader gives meaning to the words. The child's aural language is really the cap on the use of context. Understanding of what is represented in print really determines how well context can be used. At a much more sophisticated level of achievement words may approach being ideograms in some contexts. For deaf readers, printed words may well have to reach the level of ideograms.

In the use of synonyms and antonyms, one helpful technique involves word lists. This is a perfectly sound procedure for a vocabulary development program in which the goal is passing a vocabulary test. It probably has very little to do with functional aspects of vocabulary. However, if passing a test means a child can advance, then educators have a moral obligation to help all children move up as far as possible.

CONCEPTS, NOT WORD LISTS

For learning disabled children who are quite bright and for average achieving children, the program recommended here is not based on word lists but on concepts. The technique works exceptionally well. For example, a concept to be elaborated might be "dividing something into parts." The children are presented with a problem such as what word they should use to mean dividing into parts when they talk about paper, cloth, steel, wood, etc. The teacher should use as many materials as possible, hoping to get words such as cut, tear, saw, rip, shear, etc. For gifted/learning disabled children, this technique might be doubly difficult, first because of the vocabulary problem itself and second because it requires them to be flexible, which is not characteristic of them.

The same fundamental procedure can be used with antonyms but is much more difficult and should be used only after the children have worked well with synonyms. In the development of antonyms, gifted/learning disabled children's problems with adaptability come to the fore. Using the above example, the children are required to think of an antonym "for dividing into parts" that fits paper, cloth, steel, wood, etc. The teacher would hope to get glued, pasted, sewed, welded, brazed, etc.

When dealing with adjectives, the use of context is required again. When discussing a lion, the color might be identified as tan but if it has some yellow in it, tawny might be more appropriate. The children can be asked to find pictures of or list the names of tawny things. They also might be asked to discover different types of tans and why they are labeled differently.

FOLLOW-UP FACTORS

In follow-up activities, a daily segment should deal with vocabulary, specifically synonyms and antonyms. For example, the children have read the following short selection:

Not all dinosaurs were huge creatures. Many of them were as small as dogs. Some were carnivorous; others were herbivorous. Some of them may have been cannibals.

A vocabulary section of the follow-up might be written. For example:

Directions: Find the words in the selection that mean the same or nearly the same as the words below. Write the words in the blanks.

gigantic _____
meat eaters _____
canines _____
beasts _____
probably were (three words) ____ ____ ____
eater of their own kind _____

For antonyms that would be more difficult, a different activity could be provided. For example:

> *Directions:* Find the words in the selection that mean the opposite of the words below. Write the words in the blanks.

small _____	large _____
none _____	vegetarians _____

It is important in such activities that the children be required to write the words. This is one more attempt at reinforcement and it also implies that they will be attentive enough to make sure the spellings are correct. Teachers should insist that the children proofread their writings against the text.

In the area of roots, the concept of affixes should be understood as an integral part. Too often, the use of Latin and Greek roots is reviewed as a meaning task. Children are taught what certain roots mean and then are asked to join them to produce meanings. They often do not succeed. Children might learn bio = life and logos = study and therefore biology means the study of life. However, they might learn photo = light and graph = write. They might never realize that a photograph is what is accomplished by a camera.

Children should learn these important Latin and Greek base words for two reasons: (1) they give an indication, often very clearly, of the basic meanings in the word, and (2) these elements should become a part of the pupils' sight recognition. Children should begin to see photo as an element and recognize that something about light is involved. However, once again, if they do not have the context and language rhythm skills, these elements are of no value and may actually be confusing.

For strong words in English, the use of affixes is a valuable technique. For example if the words "break" and "know" are used, the teacher can supply a number of affixes. The children are required to attach the affixes, determine whether they are appropriate, and then what the new words mean. The use of this technique on a regular basis can develop recognition and understanding. For example:

> *Directions:* Use the words break and know. Add prefixes un-, non-, im- and the suffixes -ible, -able.
> Try to form words, check to see whether each is a word and, if it is, write its meaning.

The teacher would look for "breakable," "unbreakable," and "nonbreakable." The question is: will the child appreciate the need for *n* on "know" to develop "unknow*n*?"

FUNDAMENTALS AND ELABORATION

In many instances the real value of the activities is in the oral/aural discussion for which they provide the source. It must be kept in mind, however, that if language facility is limited, extreme care is necessary in using these techniques to develop fundamental language ability first, with elaboration of ability as a later goal.

Compound words are considered to be a part of vocabulary development in many programs. The same criticism applies to this idea that was mentioned in regard to the Latin and Greek base words and roots: simply putting two words together to form another word does not always work. If a fireplace is a place for a fire, is a firehouse a house for a fire? It should be remembered that compound words actually are an element of word recognition. To have this process work effectively, children must recognize at sight the words that make up the compound word and then relate it to the context and their own past experience. It is very difficult to assign this procedure to the development of vocabulary, since it is most clearly a word recognition technique.

Vocabulary development must be a part of everything that is being done to help gifted/learning disabled children to develop. When the programs described in this text for classification skills, levels of abstraction, and relevancy are followed, one of the outcomes must be greater language facility and a larger, broader vocabulary.

It is vitally important that the teachers of these children keep in mind multifaceted development. A number of tasks must be accomplished for each activity. Since language is the major element in all activities, language and vocabulary development should always be one of the goals of a specific skills-oriented program.

SUMMARY

In summary, the vocabulary program should be realistic in light of the needs of gifted/learning disabled children. Emphasis needs to be placed on broadening their vocabulary but a program in deepening the vocabulary of certain children is necessary for diagnostic purposes.

If they develop facility in the use of context, then subtleties of language might be fostered. However, this goal may have to be abandoned for some. In such a situation, teachers must be aware of these youngsters' literal approach to words and guard against verbal subtleties in communicating with and instructing them.

There should be vocabulary development activities of an independent nature each day; these often should be the source of direct personal interaction to foster vocabulary growth.

Care should be taken to make certain that any commercially prepared (as opposed to teacher designed) vocabulary development materials really are worthwhile. Do they do what they say they do? These materials should have construct validity as much as tests should, since, in effect, in many cases they are tests first of all.

Vocabulary development cannot be left to incidental learning or independent reading. There is far too much to learn for learning disabled children, even if they are gifted.

Part IV

Written Language Unit

It is in the area of written language that many gifted/learning disabled children are discovered. Schools have subordinated writing to reading for a number of decades so problems in this language ability seldom are evaluated. Spelling difficulties are discovered but the whole spectrum of skills involved in writing often is ignored. Unfortunately, for many children discovery comes too late for remediation, and the necessity for adaptation arises. This unit deals with the development of writing ability from a remedial and adaptive standpoint.

Chapter 13

Remediation Procedures for Written Language

The field of written language has received little attention in a formalized sense for a number of decades. Because of the drive for accountability, especially in reading, emphasis shifted from language development to reading. Materials and tests required less and less writing since numbers, letters, and lines could be used to indicate answers. The pressures of class size and student numbers precluded attention to writing since the resulting papers had to be handled individually and required more of teachers' time than was considered appropriate.

During the decades of the 1960s and 1970s a trend was apparent in society to regard feelings as more valuable than words. Music, especially with a strong beat, became more important than lyrics. Whether the deemphasis on writing brought this phenomenon about or, conversely, whether it led to the deemphasis on writing is a moot point. It is apparent that written language has been in a state of decline.

The explosive growth of electronic devices also played a part in the denigration of writing. It became common for individuals to communicate through exchanged tape cassettes. During the Vietnam conflict this type of communication, which admittedly is more personal, came into extensive use. Parents and college students carried on taped conversations in lieu of writing letters. College classrooms blossomed with tape recorders.

Possibly as an unfortunate consequence of the confluence of these different trends, another troublesome development arose: children genuinely disabled in this area remained unidentified for too many years. The time in which remediation could have been effected, but never was, can never be retrieved. It is apparent that once a child reaches puberty, the degree of remediation possible becomes more and more limited and the amount of self-confidence declines.

The author, in personal experience, has seen the heartbreak in school systems across the country because the writing difficulties of very bright children have gone undetected. In many cases the awareness of the problem was not evidenced until senior high school. Gifted young people are being excluded from college or must seek special schooling because of this problem. Many with superior intelligence are not attempting to enter college since they cannot face the burden or shame of writing disability.

THE PHILOSOPHY OF WRITING

For many of the problems in writing, especially for learning disabled children, there are solutions; for others, adaptive techniques may be the only answer. (See Appendix 6-G, on developmental, remedial, and adaptive procedures.) To make a reliable decision on these matters, detailed diagnostic procedures might be necessary but it is possible that diagnostic observation and teaching might be all that is required. The services of a clinical psychologist or neurologist might have to be requested if it appears that general educational procedures have not been effective or enlightening.

The process of writing also should be analyzed as a system in the same manner as reading, which has been dissected in so much detail. This concept is important because of its psychological thrust. The elements of the procedure must be brought into prominence. In many situations writing has been looked upon as written spelling, with its base in oral spelling.

The process of writing also must be viewed from its place in the language development sequence, not as an entity apart from all the others. One of the dangers in a systems analysis of writing is the same as what has happened in reading: individual subsystems are treated in isolation and the dynamics involved are forgotten. If the sequence of language development is kept in the forefront of educational planning, this danger should not be of concern.

Therefore, to deal with problems in producing written language, educators must recognize that it is a complex, multifaceted behavior and that it must be viewed as one component of the acquisition of language functions.

THE WRITTEN LANGUAGE SYSTEM

As with reading, an analysis of the writing process can become so detailed as to become meaningless from an educational point of view. Many aspects of language are inherent in the word acquisition process and do not appear to require real cognitive effort. These, of course, could be determined, but to little avail for teaching.

In a less complex fashion, writing can be said to have six subsystems. Three of these are:

1. grammar: the relationships of words to each other to provide a meaningful pattern

2. syntax: the relationship of words to each other in a sentence to convey ideas
3. composition: the structuring of sentences to provide a modified message

It must be noted that these three are based on and are required aspects of spoken language. It does not seem feasible that gifted/learning disabled children could not learn these skills orally but could practice them in writing.

The three other subsystems of writing are:

1. spelling: the agreed-upon sequence of letters that constitutes an accepted word
2. handwriting: the means by which the letter sequences are recorded
3. punctuation: the use of certain signs to indicate in written language the elements of intonation that occur in oral language but cannot be recorded in print

These three aspects are indigenous to the writing process and usually are acquired in school. There is nothing inherently human in these processes since vast civilizations have existed that never required them for greatness. However, in today's civilization, certain aspects of life require writing; success, at least in most cases economic success, cannot be achieved without it. (See Appendix 6-I, on literacy and its varied aspects.)

EVALUATION PROCEDURES

It does not appear possible to do an adequate job of evaluating writing on the basis of available standardized tests. An informal appraisal would seem to be better In fact, a detailed case study approach involving standardized measures, especially of intelligence, informal procedures, and diagnostic observation and teaching, may be the best method of all.

A very satisfactory technique is to obtain from the child or youth written language samples of three different types—narration, description, and exposition—but not using those terms. The teacher should discuss with the writer in detail what the samples should include. This phase of the evaluation can easily be handled with a small group.

When the samples are returned, they are analyzed on the basis of the six written language aspects discussed earlier. The teacher should note particular problems in any or all of the areas and share the findings with each student individually. At this time, total evaluation, grades, happy faces, etc., should be avoided. These samples should be guidelines for meeting student needs.

It is helpful to have a 5″ × 7″ card for each child. The teacher lists the specific skills that need improvement under each of the six areas analyzed. On the basis of these cards, small groups with a common need can be formed and as children begin to show mastery of certain skills they can be allowed to scratch out the problems. It is important to be as specific as possible about the needs demonstrated. It is more helpful to recognize the need for control of plural endings than to address the generalized statement of problems with endings.

The initial concentration should be on the three total language components: grammar, syntax, and composition. If appropriate, the writing effort can begin in an oral language program to develop standard English. It is of little avail to worry about punctuation, spelling, etc., if the grammar, syntax, and composition are not suitable for sharing with others. The teacher must always keep the children thoroughly aware that they write to express their ideas to others. It is their responsibility to prepare their writings in such a way as to accomplish this task.

Evaluation of spelling provides a dilemma. Two spelling evaluations are possible: the ability to recite the successive letters of a word orally and/or the ability through a motor act to print out in some fashion the successive letters of a word. These obviously are different but that difference is neglected too often in evaluations.

Since writing is the goal, the first evaluation should be of written spelling. There ought to be at least two fundamental evaluations: (1) with the writing examples suggested earlier, and (2) with the conventional graded word list type of evaluation. In both, the types of errors should be noted precisely.

The use of standardized spelling tests should be questioned for children with reading and writing problems. In nearly all of these tests the usual procedure involves student recognition of the correct form of a word among four distractors. The diagnostic worth of this procedure is minimal for children with severe problems. However, with achieving children, these tests can be of value since they measure the last aspect of writing words—proofreading. Good writers usually do not regard words as misspelled, they usually "don't look right." A person who has reached this stage is extremely unlikely to have a disability in this area.

Once the teacher has made either or both of these evaluations, the results should be analyzed in another way. All words that were misspelled or, better, miswritten, should be dictated to the child for oral spelling. This is an effective way to determine whether the error was caused by a lack of knowledge of the letter sequences or an inability to record them correctly with a motor response. For many gifted/learning disabled children, handwriting is the operative problem but since no analysis is made beyond the written spelling evaluation, programs in spelling are provided that do not meet the primary need.

If it is apparent that the oral and written spelling are basically the same, then the child's learning technique must be analyzed. This can be accomplished by assigning two or three words to study, then analyzing the child's behavior. There may be evidences of oral spelling unrelated to writing, sounding-out procedures that are too inaccurate, or rote techniques that are of no consequence. Evaluations of memory span also can provide clues to failure if letter-by-letter learning is tried and the child's memory span proves to be very short.

If there are pronounced motor difficulties, handwriting instruction might best be minimized. If motor problems do not seem to be a cause, then formal handwriting instruction can be helpful.

The possibility of an adaptive device also should be explored in evaluating word writing. After the written and oral spelling have been evaluated, the child should be given an opportunity to type some of the miswritten words. These results then are analyzed in light of the other outcomes.

Based on these evaluation procedures, the teacher should write a report that includes as much precise information as possible. Any suggestions for remediation or adaptation should be within the teacher's capability of implementing. The report and its recommendations should be shared by the teacher, parents, and child.

INSTRUCTIONAL PROGRAM

Difficulties in grammar and syntax often are not problems in a true sense. As a vehicle for communication at home and in the community, nonstandard English must be considered correct since it tends to involve effective face-to-face communication.

However, children must understand that written language is not used often for face-to-face exchanges but is relied on for delayed communication. Therefore, the reader must be able to understand the writer.

Standard and Nonstandard English

As early as possible, children must be taught to be aware that language is a social tool that fits or does not fit certain situations. Good or bad language per se does not exist. Children must learn that one type of language is appropriate in one situation but may not be in another. The appropriateness is based on whether the language has been effective. The emotional reactions of people who teach standard English to children who use nonstandard English seem to rest on this understanding. Nonstandard English is effective in certain situations. However, it is useless to write in that style to those who cannot use it. The corollary also is true: Can someone who understands only nonstandard English be expected to comprehend materials written in standard English? It is doubtful and may well account for depressed achievements in reading and other academic areas by socioeconomically deprived children who typically use nonstandard English for oral communication. Language is either effective or ineffective, not good or bad. Any value judgments about language must be based on its effectiveness, not on the purity of a single language form concept.

Teachers who work on grammar and syntax problems must develop the concept of the effectiveness of language with the children and their parents and, unfortunately, with some fellow teachers. No one should ever be able to accuse a teacher of denigrating a child's language. The positive approach can be accomplished only if an overall philosophy toward language effectiveness is developed first.

With the following language experience approach that has been found useful, the teacher should:

- develop a reading chart with the children and, if necessary, accept nonstandard English
- rewrite the chart in standard English, once success in reading the chart has been demonstrated; introduce the idea of *book talk*—the way language is used in texts
- assure the children that both charts are useful but that the second is the way they must be written for everyone to understand
- ask the children deliberately, during the writing of subsequent charts, whether or not they are book talk; pick out specific grammatical or syntactical problems
- ask the children, as they develop recognition, to construct a chart in book talk from the beginning
- provide reading matter written in both forms and ask the children to identify each
- use regular print media and have the children pick out elements in standard English for which they might have a nonstandard version

As this procedure is followed with a group, more specific problems that are detected can be handled with work sheets or commercially prepared materials. However, in all of these materials it is important to work toward goals that are short range, attainable, and measurable. If the evaluation and recording processes suggested earlier are used, this presents no problem in organization for the teacher and provides the children with the satisfaction of progress they can perceive.

It should be evident that grammar and syntax problems, if they are extensive, cannot be resolved quickly. However, if the instructional program is truly integrated in all language areas, oral and written, then a more rapid and more effective resolution can be expected than with nonintegrated, isolated instruction.

Analysis of Composition

The analysis of composition is quite important for the learning disabled child, gifted or otherwise. Certain characteristics should receive special scrutiny:

- Are the thought patterns disjointed because of failure to use time factors (a strong characteristic of learning disabled children) or is the disjointed pattern the result of assumed understandings that a reader might not appreciate (often a characteristic of gifted children)?
- Is the vocabulary that is used generally correct but inappropriate in the context and is there a tendency to use the same terms repeatedly, since gifted children with writing handicaps often express themselves in this fashion?
- Are words omitted from written sentences not because of faulty spelling or carelessness but because of simple failure to perceive the omissions? One or two instances of such behavior probably are not significant but a larger number might indicate a learning disability. If this tendency toward omissions is a standard operating procedure for the child, this too might be indicative of a true learning disability.

Caution is necessary at this time. It must be kept in mind at all times that writing follows reading in the sequence of language development. It also is important to appreciate that writing as a process is more than simply recorded talking. Therefore, the child who has had problems learning to read or has not achieved well for whatever reason brings to the writing situation little to draw upon. Success in written composition relies to a marked degree on models with which the child has come in contact—the writings of others. If there have been no models available, the first procedure may simply be to provide them. This, of course, means that achievement in reading would be a prerequisite to success in writing.

The need for composition models is just as important for grammar and syntax. The language experience approach is an ideal vehicle for instruction because:

- It is a sound technique for developing reading ability.
- It provides a teacher with the opportunity to juxtapose written-down talk and written expression.
- It provides an opportunity to develop standard English concepts of grammar and syntax during the dictation part of the procedures and, if necessary, when the transfer from written-down talk to book talk is being carried out.

The modeling procedure needs to be augmented in another way. On a daily basis, even for limited periods of time, children should be read to. This is an excellent supplement for those who have not had enough success in reading to relate to the writing models. This procedure does carry with it benefits other than development of writing models. For some children it may be their first contact with the joys of the printed page and through such reading they may acquire and process new information. (See Appendix 6-B, on directed listening activity.) Finally, there is the aspect so important for gifted children—the arousing of new interests. Instructional processes can be further integrated as an outgrowth of reading to children.

Integration of Language

It is evident that the improvement of the nonindigenous aspects of the writing process cannot be accomplished without overall language integration.

For the indigenous aspects there is a fundamental integration of skills that is of paramount importance. The need is to recognize that words are written. It is important to keep in mind that oral and written spelling are two different behaviors and in effect there is very little use or value in oral spelling outside of school. Yet in many school systems and homes, spelling is considered writing. The lack of recognition of writing as a language function could well be traced to this faulty perception.

An important adjustment that teachers should make is to eliminate the term "spelling" when helping children with writing skills. Words should be written; errors should be noted as not written correctly, or as miswritten. A serious effort must be made to help the children avoid a letter-by-letter approach to writing.

Spelling Remediation

Remediation of spelling problems has always been a controversial issue. The problems are multifaceted. Spelling often is viewed as the converse of reading and therefore is based on phonic skills. Others feel that rote memorization of letter sequences, orally or in writing, is necessary. However, these programs always require recitation of letter names in sequences. Still others view spelling as a syllabic activity and believe that the written syllable must be reinforced, with no letter names or sequences required, as suggested in Appendix 6-C.

This last concept is the one endorsed for this writing program. It also is advocated for all learning disabled children, not only those who are gifted. It is presumed that writing is not the converse of reading. Reading can be considered an auditory-visual activity while writing is auditory-kinesthetic. Individuals write with their hands, and no vision is required. Words can be written (and spelled correctly) in the dark or with the eyes closed. Print cannot be read that way.

The Instability of Phonics

It also seems rather simplistic to expect such an unstable system as phonics to be successful. Many individual graphemes can represent a large number of phonemes. It is even more perplexing to hear of children having much difficulty learning to read through an intensive phonics approach yet using this same procedure to solve a writing disability.

In a textbook for teachers of learning disabled children, one task for the instructor was to determine whether the children could hear the ending sound "s." Two of the words used were tusks and eyes. Both end in "s" but the sounds at the ends of the words are, respectively, "s" and "z." A child with good phonics skills in writing should then write the word eyes incorrectly. It requires only a little time working with phonetics and phonics to find numerous instances where the sound-symbol system fails.

Memory Span Difficulties

Another problem in spelling is memory span. Most learning disabled children have trouble in this area. Often they cannot repeat four meaningful words immediately after hearing them. Is there any wonder why letter-by-letter spelling fails them even with the addition of kinesthetic reinforcement? Most people cannot remember ten digits in a memory span test but can repeat them if they are administered as three groups of three plus one by itself.

For these reasons, it is suggested that the spelling program for all learning disabled children follow the procedures discussed in Appendix 6-C on a modified Fernald Procedure for word learning and Appendix 6-D on the writing activity. For gifted children, these procedures are best implemented through materials in which they have high interest and strong background. These materials strengthen recall.

It must be remembered that spelling is a recall proposition while reading is a recognition process. This distinction usually is overlooked in regular as well as remedial writing programs. For many of the children whose disability is primarily in the writing area, the addition of kinesthetic and tactile stimulation is vital even though these may be totally unnecessary in the reading process. Recognition might well be superior to recall in these children.

Some children's inability to write may be based on motor recall problems. They do know the correct letter sequences and they know when a word does not look right but the handwriting process intrudes negatively and they make incorrect reproductions.

TWO REMEDIAL SUGGESTIONS

In this situation there are two possible remedial solutions:

1. Kinesthetic and tactile stimulation, as suggested earlier, can remediate this difficulty to a large degree for some of these children.
2. Many children, but, more importantly, older children and youths, can begin to face and handle the writing situation more confidently and successfully if a typewriter can be substituted for handwriting.

If a typewriter is to be involved, common sense must be used. Conventional touch typing may be out of the question for a child with motor difficulties. The use of index fingers for "journalism" typing should be accepted and even taught. This is just as true whether the keyboard is on a typical typewriter or on a computer. (See Appendix 6-H, on the role of computers.)

Certain conditions must be observed if these suggested changes are to be successful. First, a system of personal shorthand must be developed for students who must take notes, and these pupils must understand that their notes must be transcribed as soon as possible. This means they must maintain strong self-discipline. A second condition is the need for excellent ability in handling context clues. These students must be able to put two and two together. They must be able to predict what would fit in a context and use their shorthand to determine exactness or suggest possibilities. (See Chapter 7 on word recognition.)

Because writing is the last of the language development sequences it naturally is involved with more accumulated functions than the others. As a result, the remediation of writing difficulties cannot be the simplistic procedure that often is offered to children with problems.

The same types of procedures that were suggested for reading retention should be used to evaluate recall in writing. There should be daily, weekly, and monthly evaluations of words learned for writing. If possible, the first check should be in isolation, a word simply dictated. The second check should involve sentence writing. It is important to note whether or not there is a change of performance in the two modes. It is hoped that the contextual writing will be better than that in isolation. However, for some children who have had drilling in spelling, the converse may be true. The rate of improvement for such children in the true sense of writing is slower and in a few unfortunate cases the prognosis for success is not good. Writing has been made so unpalatable so often that emotionality—fear, withdrawal, etc.—overrides any real chance for learning to occur. (See Chapter 14, on developing proofreading.)

Of course, a few children and youths are so disabled that the remediation procedures suggested will be of no avail. They can operate at only the lowest functional writing level. Adaptive procedures may be the only means available for dealing with their problem. The difficulties lie in the adult world of schools. It is a dreadful loss to society when creativity is dissipated because an individual cannot write. This type of person needs to be able to take examinations orally and to prepare term papers and reports on a tape recorder.

Far too frequently these adaptations are considered unfair concessions and are not permitted. Some authorities seem to feel that if a child does not behave exactly as do all the others, the rewards must be diminished. Some educators regard these adaptive devices as unfair to other children. It appears that all children must pay the same dues. Some major authorities in different fields dictate their materials for a secretary to type, yet their credentials as producers of worthy publications never are challenged. One wonders how long these constraining authorities can continue to fight off the challenges of the electronic revolution.

THE PUNCTUATION PROBLEM

Punctuation as the last of the indigenous skills presents an interesting area for analysis. Punctuation is a nearly perfect example of the literacy problem. One aspect is functional: initial and proper name capitalization and final punctuation. The other aspect is rather sophisticated: the use of effective internal symbols. The more sophisticated aspects often even go through vogue phases—commas are in or out, semicolons and dashes rise and fall, etc.

For children with writing problems, the functional aspect must be dealt with first. It permits their writing to be correct, if not sophisticated, which relieves home and school pressures. A detailed analysis of needs for all of the concepts in this area should lead to the pinpointing of specific requirements. One need should be dealt with at a time. If a child does not use end punctuation, the instructor should teach the period and go on to the question mark only when the period is mastered. This step-by-step process is essential for children with writing problems or handicaps.

Growth in the appreciation and use of the more literary components of punctuation comes about as overall sophistication in language processes develops. This means that all the language functions need to be at a rather high level, and it is at that point that many gifted/learning disabled children founder. It will be recalled that there are at least three types of literacy—basic, functional, and stratified. (See Appendix 6-I on literacy.) Many of these children, because of their intense personal interests, will never really develop a literary flair. They will not be storytellers or screen writers. They will want and need to be technical writers. There is no reason why they cannot approach punctuation from a stratified point of view. They will need to be able to punctuate if they are to express effectively the ideas they are trying to convey.

SUMMARY

Schools must be able to accept the concept that gifted children might never become "Renaissance men." This same acceptance must be accorded to gifted children who are learning disabled. This acceptance can mean a totally different change of attitude by the child and probably a vastly improved set of behaviors.

The remediation of a written language disability might well be the most difficult type of corrective assistance since success depends on so many other learnings that must have been acquired as prerequisites. It cannot be broken down into minute steps that then are treated as isolated segments. The systems analysis approach must always recognize which factors impact positively and negatively on these children. Therefore, educators must look at the entire process while dealing with any of its parts.

Chapter 14

Developing Proofreading

The ability to proofread is often looked at and treated as if it were innate. However, it is something that must be learned and, therefore, can be taught. The fundamental problem in this area is psychological. For an ability to be acquired, there must be a need for it. If the need does not exist, proofreading will not be learned. Therefore, the first aspect of instruction in proofreading is creating the need.

The need is best developed as a fundamental part of the written language program. Too frequently, proofreading is included as an aspect of the reading program where, of course, there is little need for it.

Interestingly, there must be adequate reading ability and appropriate attitudes about reading before the problems of proofreading development can be addressed.

The writing process, as noted in Chapter 13, can be analyzed into six major subsystems—grammar, syntax, composition, spelling, handwriting, and punctuation. Proofreading must concern itself with at least five of these areas; from the proofreading point of view, handwriting merges with written spelling.

A DEVELOPMENTAL ABILITY

It is obvious that the basic reading and writing skills and attitudes must be known before they can be applied; therefore, proofreading instruction must follow these other areas. The implications of this concept are that proofreading instruction must be planned as a regular developmental ability and must be introduced when the appropriate readiness has developed. To proofread for grammar and syntax, children must know those elements correctly. In proofreading for composition, they must read for meaning and be aware when it is not present. They must understand the correct spelling of the words and the function of the punctuation marks being proofread. Once again, the dichotomy between general language abilities and indigenous writing skills is evidenced. (Before inaugurating a proofreading program, teachers should read Chapter 7, "A Program in Word Recognition.")

A proofreading program should begin in the area of meaning. The teacher should:

- provide a number of meaningful and meaningless sentences, then have the children note those that are meaningless and state why
- have the children correct all possible errors
- note meaninglessness in their writings by indicating only that something does not make sense; insist that they proofread their materials
- insist that all materials be proofread before being turned in

These same basic procedures should be used for problems with grammer and syntax. However, the teacher must be sure that only one skill is being worked on at a time. Once all these aspects have been presented, the teacher begins to provide sentences with mixed errors. As skill with sentences is demonstrated, children begin to use a paragraph and then a number of paragraphs. Special efforts must be made with those who do not carry the meaning across paragraphs. In some instances, gifted/learning disabled children isolate ideas and paragraphs and produce a meaninglessness whole although individual paragraphs might be considered correct.

The role of meaning is paramount for skills in writing and proofreading that are based fundamentally on oral language ability. However, for spelling and punctuation skills, meaning is still important but written language axioms must be mastered as well.

SIGHT VOCABULARY THE KEY

Proofreading training for spelling is absolutely dependent on the child's sight vocabulary. This is the stock of words recognized immediately, almost as if no cortical activity is required. These words provide the standards against which legitimate comparisons are made. For example, is this word, *neoteny*, written correctly? If you have read the word previously you might know, but if you have never seen it before, you cannot know. In fact, you cannot even know whether that group of letters is a word until you take some other course of action, such as consulting someone or looking in a dictionary. In essence, you cannot proofread that word because you do not recognize its correct or incorrect form.

Because of this factor, the spelling program for gifted/learning disabled children should grow out of their stock of words developed as a part of the reading and writing programs. Interest and usefulness are maintained in this fashion. It is realistic to expect adequate proofreading from the children.

General spelling demands are made on many learning disabled children before they have developed reading ability. As a consequence, many of them demonstrate writing difficulties that are not genuine disabilities. When these children are provided with a systematic approach to reading, writing, and proofreading, many of these so-called disabilities disappear. This factor is one more reason why remedial education must concern itself with short-range, attainable goals.

PUNCTUATION AND MEANING

Proofreading for punctuation must follow the written language instructional program. Again, the first elements stressed are capitalization of the first word in a sentence and the proper nouns, followed by work on the final punctuation elements. The first elements can be approached using simple visual recognition skills. However, as soon as proper nouns and final punctuation become the focus of instruction, the use of meaning must be reemphasized.

This meaning aspect also must be highlighted when proofreading internal punctuation is introduced. Some aspects such as the recognition of the use of a colon with a series or of a semicolon as a conjunction often are taught as routines yet when children are faced with the need to proofread, their lack of real understanding is evidenced by their failure to recognize either a need or an error. If this more demanding stage of development is reached, teachers should feel encouraged because remediation has occurred with the less complex elements.

This may never be a goal for many learning disabled children, especially gifted ones. Because of their tendencies to be highly selective in their interests and goals, many of the gifted/learning disabled need a stratified written language program, since the reading program probably will be stratified also. The proofreading program of necessity would then have to conform to this stratification.

However, for gifted/learning disabled children whose disabilities are primarily in written language, especially written spelling, good adaptive procedures might well allow them to attempt many types of written literacy. Of course, they should be provided with all that is necessary to foster satisfactory proofreading. Typing and adult and peer dictation can be very helpful.

Gifted children who are disabled in writing may have so much emotionality involved in the program that limited types of literacy may be a teacher's only recourse. Withdrawal and rebellion are not unheard of. It is hoped that the proofreading program parallels as nearly as possible the skills developed in the written language program. The school system may even demand it.

In many remedial programs, proofreading is virtually ignored. Inabilities in this field can have a devastating effect. Many young people who believed they had been remediated enter regular programs, especially freshman year in college, with high hopes. Failure in all subjects requiring written composition occurs and personal failure is reintroduced. For many of these students, ideas and composition are not the cause of failure; their inability to submit adequately and satisfactorily prepared materials is. It is interesting to note how frequently these students did not recognize the inadequacy of their work.

Proofreading is not an innate ability. It must be taught and learned in a systematic fashion. For gifted children whose disabilities in written language go undetected too long, this ability takes on particular significance.

Part V

Supportive Aspects Unit

An instructional program per se theoretically might be extremely effective yet fail for the learners because certain necessary philosophical, administrative, and ancillary components were not in place for the effort to be a success. This unit deals with some of those components that appear to be very important in dealing with learning disabled children, especially those who are gifted.

Chapter 15

The Learning Experience

Throughout this text the need for a systematic learning experience has been a common thread. All children need this approach, learning problem youngsters even more so, and gifted problem learners need it especially in certain components.

It is assumed that learning is an orderly process and, therefore, the instruction should be orderly to mesh with the learning. There are four important components of the learning experience:

- teaching or independent behavior: in this aspect, the knowns that the learners will need are either presented or contacted
- reinforcement: in this activity the knowns are dealt with repeatedly to ensure retention because repetition breeds retention
- enrichment: in this area, new retained learnings are linked to old learnings to promote recall
- applications: in this field, concepts, vocabulary, and skill elements now available to the learner are put to regular use

These are the fundamental requirements of any curriculum dedicated to fostering learning.

In the teaching component, the most important factor is teacher decision. Teachers must decide which concepts, vocabulary, or skills are to be learned, then provide the necessary percepts. This is the stage in which criterion-referenced inventories and teacher observations and judgments come into play. It is where teachers of the gifted/learning disabled must be freed from nonflexible school system guides and programs. Teacher creativity and sophistication are crucial. Instructors must be able to see in the interests and backgrounds of the children the percepts that can become the basis for academic progress. Routine-bound teachers usually do not recognize or appreciate these opportunities.

Repetition is the fundamental ingredient in retention. It also is the fundamental problem with slow learners, although it is often not recognized. Many learning disabled children have strong elements of slow learning in their behavior. This is just as true of the gifted/learning disabled but because they are intelligent, this particular handicap often is overlooked, with resultant unsatisfactory programming. The amount of repetition needed varies from individual to individual and in each person it varies from type of learning to type of learning. Words may take more repetition than numbers for some children, or vice versa. This factor often goes undetected when evaluations and diagnosis are made.

Enrichment is the key factor in promoting recall. It is easier to recall things that have been related to things that already have been learned. Many of the so-called memory improvement programs are based on this proposition. For certain children, especially those from impoverished backgrounds, this is the root of their learning problem. They are so limited in their backgrounds of experience that new learnings may well be retained but be unavailable for recall.

With some gifted children it is possible that some of the same problems can occur because they can become enmeshed in a very limited or exotic interest area. Those who teach these types of children need to focus on this interest initially until a broadened background has developed. Even if the backgrounds are broad and diverse, it must be remembered that new learning always should be integrated with these backgrounds. This is one of the many reasons why "canned" remedial programs often fail for gifted/learning disabled children.

The element called applications is necessary for two major reasons:

1. Applications tell the children that, in contradiction to many of their former experiences, what was taught and learned was important. This is a vital point to be made to many gifted students who have seen little or no value in what they were taught. The need for relevancy of curriculum and materials has been and is being debated but for many gifted children it has become a dead issue. Their experiences have led them to the negative idea that much of what is involved in schooling is useless.
2. The fundamental human reaction of forgetting also is significant. Most people with college degrees had to learn to balance chemical equations, yet today most of them could not. The reason is basic. Humans do not clutter their minds with useless procedures. They slough off useless things. If children are expected to use learned materials, periodic application is necessary.

The four elements of the learning experience developed here are essentially time oriented. Immediately after teaching, retention activities should be provided. At a later time, once it is thought that retention has occurred, enrichment activities should be introduced. After recall has been demonstrated, periodic application should be provided.

It is important to note that prediction of retention is always intuitive. Retention can be measured only by recall procedures. This means that things recalled have been retained but not that unrecalled material has not been retained. Children may know something but be unable to recall it. This phenomenon is called "having something on the tip of your tongue." It is not that something is not known; it is just that it cannot be recalled at the moment. Because of the intuitive aspect of recognizing retention, teachers need time to get to know students' reaction patterns so that after a few experiences they can begin to step up their activities with the children at the most profitable rate.

For ideas on the implementation of this concept, see Chapter 17 on classroom management procedures.

Chapter 16

The Teacher As a Learning Therapist

In nearly every discussion or presentation on learning disabilities, the factor of emotional disturbance or adjustment difficulties is sure to arise. In most cases, discussing emotional components of learning disability is itself an emotional issue. Factions have developed with very strong points of view.

One faction that appears to be unrealistic, if honest diagnostic observation is employed, states that children may have learning disabilities with no negative emotional overlay. There is a group of educators and a large segment of parents who espouse this idea. As noted earlier, there is comfort in this idea since it relieves educators or parents of any blame for causing the problems. Many school systems also accept this point of view, which is unfortunate since it precludes the necessity for their providing services to the emotionally handicapped.

Another faction accepts the factor of emotional disturbance along with learning disability. As is often the case, a dichotomy exists in this faction. One group feels that the emotional problems are basically the cause of the disability; the second is the reverse, ascribing the emotional problem to the disability and its lack of recognition and treatment.

The major proponents of these two points of view are rather obvious. Educators on the whole tend to see the child coming to the learning situation and being unable to profit from it because of emotional factors in the home. For many gifted/learning disabled children this may well be true. On the other hand, parents often feel that the emotional problems developed because an appropriate educational program was not provided. This undoubtedly is true for many gifted/learning disabled children. However, in reality, the two positions are probably not even worth debating.

From experience, it seems clear that by the time a child with learning problems reaches second grade in a conventional school, emotional factors must begin to surface. Withdrawal, acting out, or sleep problems may appear. At that point,

whether the problems were brought to school or arose there is of little consequence. The problems have been so intertwined that dealing with only one
accomplishes little. This recognition must be accepted by administrators and
parents if the teacher is to operate as a learning therapist.

CHARACTERISTICS OF LEARNING THERAPISTS

Teachers as learning therapists need certain personal qualities and professional
attitudes. They need resiliency. In effect, they must be able to roll with the
punches. They must be able to accept the variability that is usual with the
gifted/learning disabled. All learning disabled children tend to have peaks and
valleys in their skills and information, the gifted ones have them higher and
deeper. It is difficult to accept an 8-year-old who can catalogue dinosaurs but does
not know the days of the week.

Teachers' resiliency seems to come when they have strong egos themselves
and, therefore, do not overly invest their egos in the children's successes or, more
importantly, their failures. Educational therapists must always keep in mind that it
is the children's responsibility to learn. The teachers must provide the best
possible place and material for the students to meet that responsibility.

Therapists also must be adaptable. Their planning must be done in light of the
children's needs. They must grasp opportunities such as television programs and
special activities, etc., when they are appropriate but not do so when the children
are not prepared to profit from them. Children's learning must not be restricted by
grade or curriculum guides. The learning therapists must be able to move in and
out of skill sequences and use curriculum topics that grow out of the interests of the
group. It is important that interests are developed and transmitted from individuals
to the group and from the group to individuals.

The learning therapists must be aware of the interaction between academic
success and failure and children's emotions. With gifted/learning disabled students, the therapists have a major responsibility in this interaction, which is the
reason for their title.

Learning therapists must keep the students aware of reality at all times. This
does not imply insensitivity or lack of understanding in problem situations. It does
mean that the denial, projection, and rationalization noted earlier as characteristics
of the behavior of gifted/learning disabled children are recognized when they
occur and are dealt with.

It is at this point that the therapists need strong egos. They must be secure as
people and as teachers. They must understand and accept the concept that children's emotional responses that appear directed toward them are usually looking at
an unhappy past or self. Therapists must never respond in kind to this emotionality—that would lead nowhere.

At all times the teachers must show understanding but not necessarily acceptance. The latter is appropriate when error or failure occurs. The children must understand that mistakes and failure are part of learning and that errors provide teachers with information that helps in teaching. Most children can come to understand this concept.

The defense mechanisms that the children use should be discussed with them although in most cases not directly. Therapists can often take emotional pressure off with a simple statement that sometimes children feel better if they tell themselves they can do something when in fact they cannot. The defense mechanism is recognized by the teacher and accepted with nothing untoward happening. The difference between a wish and a lie is noted. Rationalization often can be handled the same way. The need for protection of the self is not considered a "bad" thing.

Projection often requires a more direct approach. At times it is simply easier to say, "Why blame someone? What good does it do? Let's solve the problem now," or "You know you miswrote the word—you control your hands." Facing up to the uselessness of blaming is vitally important. It is in this area that acceptance may need to be tempered by direct interpretation of the behavior by the teacher.

Learning disabled children must face reality at any time it is appropriate for their growth. It is even more important to have the basically good intelligence of gifted disabled students directed toward reality rather than toward fantasy. The concept behind the title educational therapist rests on the adult's sensitivity in knowing when and to what degree to require children to face reality.

PROBLEMS WITH BEHAVIOR

One of the most difficult aspects of gifted/learning disabled children's reaction systems is their passive-aggressive behavior. It is easy for teachers and parents to follow procedures that simply reinforce the behaviors. Such behaviors can be seen in many forms. One child may simply look straight ahead and not establish any eye contact. Another may simply refuse to do something. One youngster even went so far as to develop an imaginary button in his stomach that could make people "disappear." These examples could be elaborated on, and more could be presented, but their essence always would be the students' passive-aggressive nature. Children thus can get what they want by doing nothing. They do not have to face unpleasant situations.

In such situations, the learning therapists cannot allow the procedure to bear fruit. It is not the place for a nondirective approach. They can use a monologue very well to analyze the behavior, since the children put themselves in the position of a captive audience. The children must understand that teachers do know the pupils can hear what is being said. The teacher-therapists should inform the children that there are alternatives and what they are. At this point it is important to present alternatives for solutions, not to try to draw them from the children. That is why being nondirective is of little value. That can only come later.

This also is the time to express some reflective ideas. The therapists should indicate verbally that they can imagine how the students feel about certain things at certain times. But it also is the time to express a positive attitude. The therapists should reprise past successes and delineate possible future ones. When dealing with passive-aggressive behavior, they must be sure positive communication is maintained. Hope must be held out. There will, of course, have to be a time when negative behaviors are discussed but that should wait until the children have shown enough emotional growth to make the negatives positives in their eyes.

Finally, therapists should never isolate a child. If for some reason a child must leave the instructional setting, teachers must be sure an adult is present and that nonthreatening human contacts are maintained. If some type of force is permitted and required, it is vital to be sure it cannot be interpreted as punitive. The therapist should assure the child that for mutual protection, "I won't let you hurt yourself or anyone else." For many aggressive children the concept that someone will protect them from their own destructive impulses is a beginning step in better adjustment.

Learning therapists face a dilemma with many gifted nonachieving children. It is almost axiomatic that a positive attitude by the therapists is the best approach when dealing with such children. As a principle, it probably is true. However, discretion in this respect is demanded with a few children. With some, the learning therapists may need to assume the role of the superego or conscience. These children have so little faith in themselves that they cannot attempt moral, ethical, or proper social decisions. The therapists need to take on that role.

After an indiscretion, the therapist might say, "How did you think I would feel about your behavior," or "Did you think I would be proud of you for doing that?" This can be done in a manner that indicates personal hurt based on caring for the child. Most pupils with this problem can begin to accept the therapists' values as a standard for behavior. In group activities, status is maintained if negative behavior is stopped because of the therapists rather than because the children are "being chicken" and backing off from whatever wrong actions they have been performing.

The dilemma occurs when a decision must be made to foster the superego skills in the children and away from the therapists. This can be addressed by offering positive reinforcement on small behaviors: "You did that well without any help from anyone," or "I'm sure you can handle that." If such comments lead to regressive behavior, then there is a clear indication that it is prudent to stay away from positive reinforcement. That should not be attempted until later. If no regressive behavior occurs, then it is safe to proceed to provide positive statements for more important behaviors, especially those that involve social interactions and responsibility for self.

It is obvious that not all teachers can become learning therapists. This is in no way a negative comment. In the life of children, many roles must be played. It is within each individual's personality that the determinants are found. If teachers can be resilient and adaptable and not feel threatened by children's failures or accusations, the role of learning therapist is available for them.

Chapter 17

Placement Procedures

The problems in dealing with gifted/learning disabled children in schools do not all center on the diagnostic or instructional programs. Some of the thorniest problems are found in placement procedures. In fact, difficulties in placement may ultimately scuttle well-intentioned diagnosis and remediation programs.

Three areas in student placement must be dealt with:

1. classroom and school placement
2. parental and community involvement
3. child involvement

CLASSROOM AND SCHOOL PLACEMENT

The major rift involving educators of the gifted—enrichment vs. acceleration—should be of no consequence when dealing with gifted/learning disabled children. Neither concept should intrude to any marked degree except for the possibility of one major unaffected area of strength, such as excellent mathematics ability, etc. In such a situation, mainstreaming to a gifted section might be appropriate.

The placement problem for gifted/learning disabled children revolves around the need for homogeneity in grouping for the pupils and the teacher. These children often feel out of place in all educational placements. In a learning disabilities class, their superior intelligence can cause them to be bored and unreceptive toward the instructional program. In some cases this is viewed as negative behavior by the other children and often by the teacher, which can further compound serious attitudinal problems.

In a gifted classroom placement, the learning disabled are confronted with their inability to do in the language arts area what their intellectual peers can accomplish. Serious problems in self-esteem and self-worth result. It does not require many such experiences for the children to develop negative behaviors and attitudes. In most respects, a learning disabilities or gifted placement leads to fundamentally the same type of diminished self-image. The real outcome of this placement dilemma is the failure of children ever to reach or approach their potential.

Even pullout programs in these special classes as a part of the mainstreaming concept usually produce the same results. The dual exceptionality—both gifted and learning disabled—always places the children in some type of jeopardy as long as the placement is based on one exceptionality.

Two possible solutions to this problem seem appropriate.

First, a teacher with the necessary training could be assigned to work with all the gifted/learning disabled in the school regardless of their age and grade. This would give the teacher a larger group for which to plan and probably less divergence for which to compensate. An important element in the education of gifted children is that they need to be helped to recognize the range of individual differences in themselves and others. It seems just as important, however, that for instructional purposes some degree of homogeneity be achieved. Bright children should profit from exposure to other bright children.

Second, if transportation could be provided, a class of gifted/learning disabled children could be formed in a given school or center. In that way the properly trained teacher could develop a classwide curriculum and instructional program that could be most advantageous to these children. Diversity of age, interests, needs, and strengths would be present but the children's ability to capitalize on these elements together would be enhanced. In such a classroom another important component of the gifted/learning disabled could be fostered. Already developed interests can be capitalized upon and new interests fostered. This could be every teacher's goal but a direct statement of it for those who instruct the gifted/learning disabled might become a credo. Horizons must be expanded.

These suggestions are, of course, counter to trends in special education and remediation of learning handicapped children. Mainstreaming has become almost a vogue. It is intriguing to note that the word "mainstreaming" never appears in Public Law 94-142, the Education for All Handicapped Children Act of 1975; instead, the law uses the term "least restrictive environment." It would be interesting to know whether, when the term was placed in the law, it was meant to be so inclusive of handicapping conditions. The goal may have been to free individuals from institutionalization rather than to promote the broad interpretation that resulted.

Far too frequently the term "least restrictive environment" has been interpreted by parents and school administrators as regular classroom placement with or without help from specialists. In many cases, both groups have seized on the term for purely adult-centered reasons.

Parents often see mainstreaming as a means of escaping the stigma of having a special education child. Too frequently this motivation is so intense that parents lose sight of the academic welfare of their child.

School administrators in a period of inadequate financial support view mainstreaming as a satisfactory way to cut costs. The use of one specialist to serve far more students than would be possible in a self-contained special education classroom is financially attractive. The possibility that there might be too little service is overshadowed by the financial relief.

Mainstreaming has been facilitated by extensive use of pullout programs. The flow is in both directions. Gifted children in learning disability classes are placed in regular classes for specific subjects, or in gifted classes. Gifted children with academic or learning difficulties are placed in special education or learning disability classrooms for instruction from specialists. Unfortunately, these arrangements in no way deal with the need for homogeneity that gifted/learning disabled children require. In many of the placements, the gifted cannot compete with their nonhandicapped peers. In the special education or learning disability placement, they face a range of handicapping conditions or lack of intellectual stimulation that is very deleterious to their progress.

In effect, these children's problems frankly are not met in most cases by mainstreaming in either direction or by pullout programs. These students need a placement that is planned to meet their needs in both exceptionalities.

PARENTAL AND COMMUNITY INVOLVEMENT

If only the students' needs had to be considered, placement procedures for gifted/learning disabled children would not be difficult. However, a number of confounding elements make placement a problem. The two most serious of these elements are parents and community.

Many parents view their children's abilities with little objectivity. In many instances they attribute to giftedness behaviors that really are only age appropriate. This is understandable, because some standard is needed to make judgments. Parents' standards, because of lack of experience with very bright children, permit them to make such inappropriate determinations.

Their lack of understanding becomes a problem in placement when they refuse to accept more valid observations and insist that others' bias and prejudice are responsible for nonacceptance of their child as gifted. In many instances educators have been known, for reasons related to politics, legalities, and convenience, to capitulate to parents on these matters, have altered requirements and standards, and at times have allowed parental recommendations for gifted placement to supersede professional criteria. In some school systems an IQ of 115 on a paper-and-pencil intelligence test is considered satisfactory for gifted placement.

Community attitudes also influence placement for giftedness but often in more subtle ways. Because the number of gifted/learning disabled children is small, community members often seek economic restraints. They question the value and even the justice of allotting money to meet the needs of these pupils. They usually contend that these students are no better than any other learning disabled children and that the learning disabilities program should be adequate for them. In many instances, the point behind this attitude is elitism. It is difficult to get a community to accept the need for justice for these children.

This same community problem exists concerning learning disabilities. Since the identification of learning disability usually requires services under the law, many school districts (in the person of their superintendent or school board) have decided that grade-level achievement is adequate. Retardation based on potential vs. achievement is left undetermined lest the learning disability be noted. This attitude of not seeking the problems makes budgeting easier, of course. However, the gifted/learning disabled children in such situations continue to be deprived of their right to strive for their utmost potential.

To prevent the injustice to these students, a public relations effort must be made based on objective data that attempt to avoid the emotions, disseminating information through community correspondence, parent-teacher associations, etc. Concerned parents and teachers could initiate this effort through local educational groups. The meaning of intelligence and learning disability should be clearly stated in meaningful terms so that an understanding develops about children who have both exceptionalities. Parents of children with or without learning problems must be reassured that their progeny will not be deprived of services because funds are allocated to provide special services for gifted/learning disabled. This can be done only if frank sharing of information is provided clearly and readily.

Parental pressure must be brought to bear on school boards and administrators. However, that can be counterproductive because too often parental pressure becomes strident and threatening, causing negative reactions. Most educators want to do what is best for children, all children. Parents of the gifted/learning disabled must be reasonable. They must be able to participate in a dialogue with those in authority and try to ascertain what their problems are. It might well happen that both parties need to act in concert with a school board or superintendent, since either acting alone might accomplish nothing. Parents must be able to appreciate the constraints under which administrators operate. The latter in turn must appreciate the parents' concerns even though at times the demands may be overemotional and totally unrealistic. Mutual good will always is more productive for the child than are divisive adversary relationships.

With a serious attempt at good will, parents who have put their ego needs before the children's problems might become sensitive to the pupils and appreciative of the professionals' difficulties. The professionals might begin to appreciate the hurt feelings of parents and their hypersensitivity while gaining an ally in the battle to obtain services for this special group of children. Community support must be forthcoming for professional educators who demonstrate that their first concern is the welfare of the children rather than currying favors with their superiors.

CHILD INVOLVEMENT

Many forces interplay in planning and carrying out any remediation program. Parents and community interact and react. School systems and their employees assess, diagnose, prescribe, and treat what they perceive are the problems. Yet in this interaction one element tends to be neglected since it usually is viewed as the medium for the interplay: the child is the unnoticed component.

In dealing with all children who have learning difficulties it is important that they participate actively in their education. This is even more important for the gifted youngsters. Most children with educational difficulties also have emotional problems. The question of which came first becomes irrelevant; both must be dealt with. The teacher must develop and assume the role of educational therapist. As noted earlier, instruction for gifted/learning disabled children must be more than a skills development program. (See Chapter 16 on the teacher as a learning therapist.)

Because of the blows to self-esteem that many of these children suffer, success is absolutely vital. This success must be readily appreciated and easily discerned. Short-range attainable goals must be set and kept before the children. Evaluation must be carried out in the same format. (See Appendix 6-D, on writing.) The children should be involved in the evaluation. Day-by-day and week-by-week comparisons should be made available. Pretest and posttest evaluations, where appropriate, should become a regular part of classroom routine.

Children also should have a part in the development of the curriculum. If possible, their personal interests should be accommodated. With the gifted/learning disabled, a strongly felt interest of a single child often can be expanded for a group activity. An important goal of the program should be the widening of interests. Bright children usually involve themselves in activities that are stimulating even if they are not personally interested in them.

Caution must be observed about pupil involvement in curriculum, however. Teachers and parents must be aware of the difference between interest and enthusiasm. Gifted children can become enthusiastic about many things simply because they are stimulating. One enthusiasm is likely to give way very quickly to another. Teachers who attempt to build programs on such attitudes find little success because the children contribute little or no real intellectual commitment. Parents often find themselves annoyed with gifted children, especially those with academic problems. The parents seize on an enthusiasm and provide time, energy, and money as a commitment to help the child progress only to have the eagerness die out in a short time. An enthusiasm tends to be short-lived; an interest tends to be sustained.

SUMMARY

Student placement for gifted/learning disabled children never has been viewed as a serious problem in most school systems. There is no need to be concerned since these pupils seldom are recognized. In a sense, no problem exists if no problem is recognized.

It is hoped that as recognition does emerge, the problem will be addressed honestly. This will not occur if the children are not kept in the forefront of all considerations. The school administration must provide at least adequate services. This implies placement with intellectual (not necessarily chronological) peers in self-contained as well as pullout programs.

Parents and community must be enlightened about these children and provide just services. This requires enhanced public relations activities and information dissemination. Adult needs, especially involving ego and finances, must be subordinated to the needs of the students.

Gifted/learning disabled children must be helped to appreciate their disabilities in light of their giftedness. Their participation in all parts of the program, especially in developing maturity, should be elicited.

If worthwhile placement is to be accomplished, direct participation by all parties involved is absolutely necessary.

Chapter 18

Classroom Management Procedures

If the learning experience is used as a planning philosophy, classrooms can be managed quite well. The fundamental approach espoused here applies to self-contained classrooms or those using pullout programs. The only difference between a program for all children and one for the gifted/learning disabled is in the composition of the instructional groups. (See Chapter 17 on placement procedures.)

Both time and space must be managed and time is the more important factor. However, time cannot be managed well if the environment is inappropriate. Therefore, in changing classroom management, the space component must be considered first.

THE FOUR BASIC AREAS

Any good instructional setting should have four distinct areas to conform to the requirements of the learning experience: instructional, follow-up, enrichment, and applications.

First, there must be an instructional area. In most conventional classrooms this is in the middle of the front wall with the children seated in a semicircle, or the whole room is addressed from that spot. There is a fundamental classroom control problem inherent in this procedure. One of the most important management mechanisms a teacher has is eye control, the ability to observe what is happening and to anticipate behaviors. If the teacher looks to the extreme left or right in this situation, certain areas of the classroom go unobserved. Sometimes this is momentary. However, if a drawn-out discussion is appropriate for one child in that position, the time could be much greater. Many unwanted behaviors could develop that would lead to classroom disruption for a far longer period. This factor must be considered seriously especially for handicapped children who might have emotional or adjustment difficulties.

This problem can be handled if teachers operate from corners and have the children sit in pie-shaped wedges. Teachers can see both the instructional group in the foreground and the entire classroom beyond. If furniture is deployed wisely, no part of the classroom is out of sight.

Second, there should be a place where the children work on their follow-up activities, especially those for reinforcement. This area should be close to the teaching center yet removed enough not to be distracting. It also should be close enough to permit the teacher to notice children there who might be having problems. These would be the areas listed as follow-up and independent areas in Figures 18-1 and 18-2.

Third, the place for the enrichment activities to stimulate recall should be close by or in the same area. It would be the same area, of course, if retention and recall activities were included in the same follow-up activity. If other materials are to be used, a distinct area can be provided for them.

Finally, there must be an applications area. This should encompass the kits, games, and gadgets that are so useful for continuous use of ideas and skills. If possible, a library area should be developed as a part of the applications concept. In Figures 18-1 and 18-2 this is the interest area. If a listening area is developed that uses a listening post, its most advantageous place is near the teaching area. This is because earphones prevent children in the listening center from being distracted by noise in the instructional area and pupils in the latter area cannot hear the recordings. Figures 18-1 and 18-2 show two examples of room arrangements developed by teachers.

As with most change, it is important not to be overwhelming. If the classroom is to be reordered, then the space should be rearranged first. The existing basic time scheduling can be carried over until the children accept the new seating arrangements.

Pupils in large group instruction can carry their chairs to the instructional area or can use carpet swatches or woven paper "sit-upons" for use on the floor. Large group discussions, viewings, or demonstrations can be carried out with this arrangement. It is better not to use the small group instructional area for these types of activities.

If the small group area maintains its integrity by being used only for that purpose, an interesting condition begins to develop: that familiar phenomenon called mind set. Children who may have been boisterous or noisy will arrive at the instructional area and get quiet. Within a short time this mind set produces a standard reaction. The children soon learn that in this area of the classroom they are supposed to listen, especially to the teacher. It is in reality the teacher's domain. For instructional purposes this mind set is an important asset toward attaining the teacher's instructional goals.

Figure 18-1 Classroom Arrangement, Example A

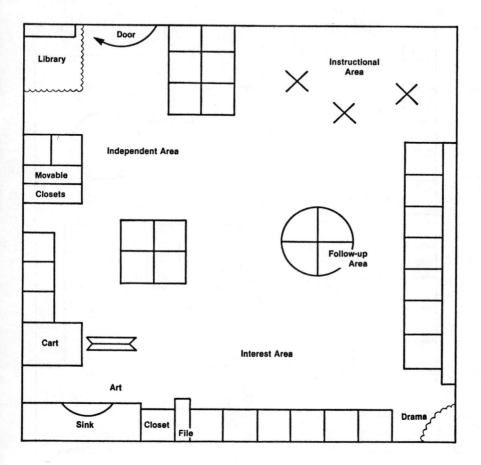

Figure 18-2 Classroom Arrangement, Example B

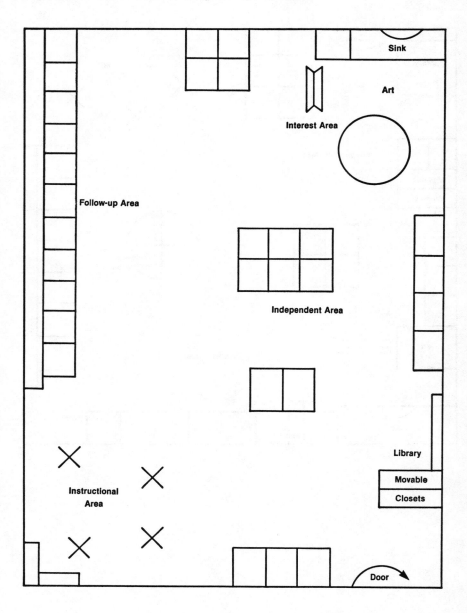

DANGERS IN CHANGES

A type of culture shock develops if care is not taken to phase in changes in the program. Instead of improved control and enhanced learning, chaos and confusion develop. If too much change is thrust on people, the original condition is more desirable even though it might have not been the most beneficial. This is just as true for children in learning situations.

This is especially important for children with learning difficulties, without regard to their intelligence. The introduction of nearly anything new causes problems. All children like and need stability but learning disabled children often seem to demand it. The children must be prepared before any program is altered and the change must be explained and as nearly as possible related to procedures and techniques that are familiar already. Gifted/learning disabled children with their tendency to lack adaptability and flexibility may well require even greater preparation for change.

It is indeed unfortunate that the effect of change, any change, on the performance of learning disabled children tends to be ignored in program planning. It never has been really pinned down whether or not educational progress is slowed down or curtailed by change. However, when children are mainstreamed in either direction or shifted from teacher to teacher or instructional group to instructional group, planned diagnostic observation should assess to some degree whether negative behavior or diminished learning is a possible outcome.

THE ROLE OF TIME STRUCTURES

Time structures are even more important than space controls in effective classroom management. Most learning disabled children, even those intellectually gifted, tend to have difficulty managing time. In fact, the inability to deal well with time and time concepts may be one major characteristic of most learning disabled children. Since time itself is so subjective, children having difficulty mastering concepts obviously will have even greater trouble dealing with the concept of time.

Therefore, it is important to provide learning disabled children with more concrete experiences that can be attached to time. The learning experience segment (Chapter 15) suggests that recall is based on attaching new learnings to old ones. That is just as true in this situation. If a child cannot appreciate the concept of a day, then a day might be related to a sleep. Morning, afternoon, and evening can be related to the appropriate meal. Unfortunately, using the converse of these procedures often does not work. It is better to address the problem as "What time of day is it when we eat breakfast?" than "What meal do we have in the morning?"

This same principle should be applied during the instructional programs. Once the space is prepared, the children should be taught the type of activity in which they are engaged, its name, and where it is to be carried out. A clearly printed schedule should always be available for the pupils to consult.

Using the learning experience as a framework, four activities should be carried out: teaching, reinforcement, enrichment, and applications, as noted at the start of this chapter. These can then be placed in a schedule for the appropriate instructional groups.

INSTRUCTIONAL GROUPS: HOW MANY?

Something must be said about the number of instructional groups a teacher manages. Most teachers who group use three sections. There has been much criticism of this, especially by those who do not have to operate in a classroom all day. There surely is nothing magical about three groups but in most cases that number is practical. More can be accomplished for children in this procedure than when a teacher tries to accommodate four or five groups. Too frequently, it is not recognized that with more than three groups the children must spend more time in independent behavior or less time in instruction. Three groups work well in terms of space usage and, as will be suggested, in time usage as well.

Time can be structured in blocks of three or four compartments, depending on the circumstances. The four-block plan called a language block in this text (Figure 18-3) provides a teacher with the opportunities to foster worthwhile instruction. This language block is based on 30-minute time segments although they can be of 20 minutes if more appropriate. Each group is provided time to engage in the parts of the learning experience.

The attitude of the groups should be considered before assigning their time schedules. Group A receives instruction first, followed by the three other activities. This arrangement implies that the group probably is the most reliable, in that its members come in ready to be taught and able to sustain themselves with minimal direction for the rest of the block.

Group B on the other hand presents a different picture because it is the most difficult one to manage. It is often suggested that this group should be worked with first when its pupils are fresh. That is often the problem. They are "fresh" in a different way—they do not want to be in school. Therefore, their first lesson could include activities less geared to academic progress. Once they have accepted the fact that they are in school, instruction can begin in the second segment, with their follow-up activity immediately afterward in the third segment. The follow-up activity usually is more structured and that area should be under the teacher's eye control. This group does not have a long, sustained period of independence because its members usually cannot handle one.

Figure 18-3 Classroom Time Structure

LANGUAGE BLOCK			
Groups	A	B	C
9:00-9:30	T.C.	I.R.	I.A.
9:30-10:00	F.U.	T.C.	I.R.
10:00-10:30	I.A.	F.U.	T.C.
10:30-11:00	I.R.	I.A.	F.U.

Key: T.C. = Teaching Center. F.U. = Follow-up Area. I.A. = Independent Area. I.R. = Independent Reading.

Group C should be the best, both academically and behaviorally. Its members must work the first hour independently and receive instruction in the third segment. If the group really is making excellent growth, the follow-up activity might be shifted to the first segment and independent activities to the fourth segment.

The teacher, in planning the schedule, should be sure that two groups are not assigned the same activity at the same time. The block provided in Figure 18-3 makes that possible.

In the fourth segment, the teacher does not teach. This is a vital aspect of classroom management and the teacher's role as learning therapist. During this time the teacher may have individual conferences, provide directions, or simply supply warm, human contact. It is time to talk of interests, new toys or dolls, new experiences, and families. It is an opportunity for the humanity in the situation to develop.

USE OF THE READING BLOCK

If it is not possible to have two hours of time or a four-segment block, then a reading block can be employed (Figure 18-4). This in essence requires the same planning as the language block except that the opportunity for teacher-children interaction is eliminated. It is suggested that once every two or three weeks the children remain at their desks during the instructional time and that the teacher use this period for personal interaction.

In the reading block format, independent activities and independent reading are combined. However, if it is thought important, this one segment could be scheduled Monday, Wednesday, and Friday for independent activities and the two other days for independent reading. The block should not be viewed as a straightjacket but rather as a structuring device.

With that in mind, there should be no reason why children could not adjust part of their schedules independently. If a pupil decides to substitute independent reading for follow-up, there should be no problem. The really crucial understanding to be developed is that whatever has been assigned must be done. When it is completed is of relatively little importance. There is one exception: the time for

Figure 18-4 More Limited Classroom Time Structure

READING BLOCK			
Groups	A	B	C
9:00-9:30	T.C.	F.U.	I.R.
9:30-10:00	F.U.	I.R.	T.C.
10:00-10:30	I.R.	T.C.	F.U.

Key: T.C. = Teaching Center. F.U. = Follow-up Area. I.R. = Independent Reading and Independent Area.

instruction from the teacher has been assigned by the teacher and can be changed only by the teacher. The other crucial element is that the follow-up must be finished before the next instruction session. Therefore, children may alter their schedules knowing that the teacher expects and demands that the follow-up will be ready for discussion and checking.

IMPACT OF PULLOUT PROGRAMS

In many pullout programs teachers find that they have only an hour with a group of children each day or for even fewer days each week. The inopportune scheduling does not mean that learning will be destroyed. In such a situation, an A-B-C schedule can be put into place (Figure 18-5). This schedule also can be employed if small group instruction is carried on in a departmentalized system at either the secondary or elementary levels.

In this schedule one of the three groups receives no direct instruction once every three days. The instructional time is divided between the remaining two groups in tandem with a follow-up activity. It is important when planning instruction in this fashion that time is always provided for the follow-up activity to be finished before the next instructional session.

This schedule does not call for any drastic revision of the space arrangement. It is helpful, however, to have an adequate supply of kits, games, gadgets, and books with enough variety to be sure that children not involved in instruction on a given day are kept meaningfully employed. These independent activities should not be thought of as busywork but as an integral part of the learning experience on which the program is based. As such, their planning and assigning should receive appropriate consideration.

Figure 18-5 Shortened Schedule for Pullout Programs

A-B-C SCHEDULE												
	First Day		Second		Third		Fourth		Fifth		Sixth	
Activity	½	½	½	½	½	½	½	½	½	½	½	½
T.C.	A	B	C	A	B	C	A	B	C	A	B	C
F.U.	B	A	A	C	C	B	B	A	A	C	C	B
I.A.	C		B		A		C		B		A	

Key: T.C. = Teaching Center. F.U. = Follow-up Area. I.A. = Independent Area.

MANAGEMENT OF MOVEMENTS

The procedures suggested in this chapter, even when well planned and carried out, are bound to cause at least minimal disruption. Teachers must keep disruption at a minimum by being systematic in their change procedures and always providing opportunities for rehearsal and practice. Great actors have rehearsals and dress rehearsals. They have readings. Yet many schools seem to assume that the children can come into new situations with new roles and not need the very techniques automatically provided for adults.

Teachers should have the children practice the movement procedures once the furniture has been rearranged, note where traffic problems occur, and decide whether they are the fault of the layout or of nonorganized passage by the pupils. If it is the furniture, it can be rearranged to solve the problem; if it is the children, they can be asked to decide what caused the problem and how it can be solved. They should suggest traffic patterns or routes to be used when changes are made in other room areas.

Once the time schedule is introduced, the children should practice the movements using very short sample time blocks—one minute and then a change. The teacher should note the problems and ask the children to do so also. They should be asked to suggest alternatives and whenever possible the teacher should use their suggestions, even though doubtful as to their success. If problems arise again, the teacher should involve the children in developing new solutions.

This routine is especially crucial for gifted/learning disabled children. It gives the teacher an excellent opportunity to provide help with adaptability and flexibility and with strong positive reinforcement. These children need to verbalize the changes, not just walk them through. The teacher's constant use of "What do you think will happen if we do that?" or "What other thing do you think we might do?" should become almost standard operational procedure in working with gifted/learning disabled children.

PROBLEMS WITH PARENTS

A new classroom management plan affects not only the children; in nearly all cases, parents become involved and often agitated, and their insecurities are heightened. Most parents know what a classroom should look like—the one they remember from their schooling. They also know why children go to school—to be taught. Therefore, they are concerned when they see a classroom in which children are not being taught and are sitting in unaccustomed (to the parents) furniture arrangements. Teachers must be aware of this problem and try to deal with it.

The first and most important step is to develop understanding. Before any changes are made, there should be an orientation program for the parents to involve them in the learning experience. The reasons for the moves, the rationale for the procedures, and the basic psychological factors behind this concept should be explained. Parents' roles in the children's programs should be delineated and encouraged. (See Chapter 21 on counseling parents of gifted/learning disabled children.)

Once again, to give credence to the program, concrete evidence of the child's activities and progress should be available to the parents. A weekly report form has been found to be especially helpful. (Figure 18-6 is a suggested form.) However, certain components should always be included. The child's name and the date the pupil receives the form should always be in the pupil's own handwriting. There should always be a place for the parent's signature. One section should provide for the child's own self-evaluation of behaviors throughout the day, with an area for teacher comments concerning that evaluation.

Another space should be provided for the child to indicate what was done in the various segments of the instructional block. These entries should include text names, page numbers covered, types of activities, names of independent activities, names of books read or looked at independently, etc. How the time was employed during the instructional block should be clearly apparent. It also is appropriate to include time references other than for instructional or independent behaviors.

Finally there ought to be a section for information concerning special areas of parental concern. A version of the form in Figure 18-6 was developed by a group of teachers in the school system in Prince George's County, Maryland. Parents in the area were particularly concerned about spelling, so words mastered were included. This section could include nearly any specific area of instruction—or more than one area.

The correct use of the form obviously is more important than the form itself. The following procedure is suggested:

- Each Monday each child is given a form and retains it for the week. The child is expected to find a place to keep it, with teacher guidance if necessary.
- Every day the children fill out the appropriate places on the form.
- Near the end of the day or instructional time, the teacher writes comments on the form.
- At the end of the week (or more often, if it seems appropriate) the children are instructed to take the form home to their parents.

At this point the effects of parent orientation or counseling should be perceived. The parents must know that a weekly report form has been supplied to the children and will be carried home. The parents have two options at this point. They may simply read it and discuss it between themselves and/or with the child or throw it

Figure 18-6 Weekly Report Form on Child's Performance

Name _____ Date _____ Group _____ Parent's Signature _____

Pupil _____   Evaluation   Teacher _____

	Mon.	Tues.	Wed.	Thurs.	Fri.
Behavior					
Work Habits					
Neatness					
Did I Finish?					
Following Plans					

Mon.	Tues.	Wed.	Thurs.	Fri.
Instruction	Instruction	Instruction	Instruction	Instruction
Follow-up	Follow-up	Follow-up	Follow-up	Follow-up
Independent Activities	Independent Activities	Independent Activities	Independent Activities	Independent Activities
Choice	Choice	Choice	Choice	Choice

My Spelling Words: _____

away. However, if they wish to discuss it with the teacher, they must sign it and have the child return it to class. This indicates a conference is requested and the teacher then can arrange one.

Some very important concepts are involved in this procedure. The children are given a responsibility for themselves and report on it to the teacher and their parents. Parents are kept informed of the program and of the child's progress and are given an opportunity to participate more fully in their offspring's education.

The procedure must be explained clearly and carried out on a regular basis. If it is handled in a haphazard fashion, nothing of value will emerge and problems may result.

SUMMARY

It is important to adjust the instructional program for children with learning disabilities even if only to indicate that there are other ways to learn and that they can profit from them.

It is even more important that any changes introduced are carried out systematically and with a clear philosophy. Changes in classroom management procedures must involve parents as well as children. These shifts should always contain as many stabilizing aspects as possible. Even gifted/learning disabled children with negative reactions to or acquiescence in change can accept it and profit from it when it grows from a genuine desire to promote their learning.

Chapter 19

Administrators' Program Responsibilities

Administrators, especially principals and supervisors, to be effective with programs for gifted/learning disabled children, do not need to be experts in either area. The important elements of their role are support and public relations.

There are two major aspects of the administrators' supportive role: support for a program and support for the teachers who staff the program. Administrators who are willing to acknowledge that gifted/learning disabled children exist in their schools must be professionally courageous because, in most cases, such explicit recognition requires financial support under Public Law 94-142. In times of financial hardship, such a move can be unpopular.

Administrators who decide that this approach is justified for these children may have to face the public charge of sponsoring elitism. These charges could be vicious enough to tear communities apart. Midlevel managers—principals, and supervisors—could have to deal with attacks from above and below. School boards and superintendents are concerned about finances and voter reactions; teachers and parents make demands about reduced loads for instructors, inadequate or unfair distribution of services, and unfortunate charges of bias and prejudice. Professional courage is indeed called for.

THE ELEMENT OF SUPPORT

Support for the teachers probably can come only if these problems are dealt with first. Teacher supports include differentiated grouping practices, permission to deviate from systemwide programs in skills and curriculum, and personalized assessment and evaluation procedures, as noted in Chapters 16 and 17.

Differentiated grouping, as noted in Chapter 18, is important for the gifted/learning disabled. The procedure of grouping them by age peers has not worked because of the polarity of their exceptionalities. Multiage and multigrade groupings are most advantageous and probably are the most difficult for administrators to authorize.

Teachers of these children must be able to seize opportunities for needed instruction whenever they develop. They also have to be able to capitalize on interests and specific bodies of knowledge. Therefore, regimentation in grade level skill sequences and curriculum spirals is not possible. Children of different ages and grades must be allowed to work on common program elements regardless of age or grade. It is in this area that conflicts with supervisors can be expected. Administrators must be able to understand the program well enough to enlist the support of other central office personnel. Comments about boat rocking from other school personnel will simply have to be accepted.

Teachers of gifted/learning disabled children must be able to operate with a high level of independence. Their principals must have confidence in them and should obtain for them the right to use tests and inventories that are not systemwide or approved. Testing and evaluations must be left to the discretion of the teachers. However, the principals should expect them to comply with systemwide standards whenever possible. The principals must demand that the right to be different also implies the responsibility to comply.

Possibly the most difficult aspect of the principals' role in such programs is scheduling. Children need time to learn. Teachers of the gifted/learning disabled must block this time through careful planning. Fragmented segments only cause problems. Therefore, in scheduling, especially for pullout programs, all these exceptional children should be scheduled with the appropriate teacher at the same time. This means block scheduling across a number of grades. Teachers of special subject matter such as physical education, art, music, etc., must adjust their programs to support the academic effort for these children.

The last support area involves teacher selection and training. In most cases the most obvious choices to work with these children are the learning disabilities teachers or the reading specialists. This approach makes sense since the disability must be overcome before giftedness can be brought to bear. However, few of the specialists noted above have any training in gifted education. This problem needs to be rectified.

A number of solutions are open to the school administration. If a teacher of the gifted is on staff, a form of modified team teaching could be planned so that the learning disabilities teacher receives some training. This is a last-gasp solution since personality conflicts could develop and the gifted teacher may be resentful. A second solution involves the use of a consultant in gifted education. In this alternative, services could be provided to teachers in the system generally but specific time and help could be made available to the learning disabilities instructors involved in the program. Money problems are a major negative factor in this alternative, as is potential grumbling from other teachers about favoritism. A third alternative involves the principal's ability to encourage the teachers to obtain training in giftedness at the university level. Implied in this alternative is the administration's commitment to support the program and provide the teachers with the elements necessary for it to work. This probably is the best solution but one that demands more than average commitment and dedication. The teachers must have enough faith in the administration to believe the necessary support will be given. They also must know that the principal will accept the role of point man. If the teachers believe they could be left in a vulnerable position with no administrative support, they cannot be expected, and rightly so, to make the necessary changes.

THE PUBLIC RELATIONS ROLE

The public relations aspect of the administrator is centered on community relations. (See Chapter 17 on placement procedures.) The public must be educated to understand the meanings of giftedness and learning disability. This is an aspect of public relations best handled by experts. Meetings should be set up to disseminate the appropriate information. It is not necessary to reach every member of the community, only the influential ones, and every principal can identify them. Child study meetings should be provided when the public can attend—perhaps several, at different hours, for various populations. Once the necessary groundwork has been laid, staff members who can explain the programs clearly and answer questions lucidly should be brought in.

In this respect, the administrator again faces a possible personnel problem. The best presenter of ideas and the most knowledgeable should participate, but the very best teacher may not have either of these attributes. It is here that the principal's human relations skills must be used. Inducing a possibly unhappy teacher to recognize that the decision was not personal but for the good of the program may take some skillful interaction but it can be accomplished.

A second aspect of the administrator's public relations effort requires the enlistment of community support without antagonizing superiors. This can produce nearly the same situation as that noted earlier with parents. Superintendents and school boards must be influenced and convinced to support programs for gifted/learning disabled children but an adversary relationship probably will not accomplish it. Parent outbursts and rudeness are inappropriate. Once again, the principal should provide difficult parents with other support and recognition while encouraging the more controlled, sensible ones to take more active roles.

Finally, with superiors, a genuine concern expressed through channels is very important. Initially, the administrator can use a conversational approach to set the scene but eventually must put something in writing to permit deliberation and decision. It is necessary to plan ahead so that decisions do not have to be rushed. The written plan should state the reasons for the program, list the outcomes and expected benefits, show how this effort will fit into the total school operation, and how it will be staffed. Whenever possible, the public relations benefits accruing to the school board or superintendent should be described. The administrator must be willing to make the commitment of time and energy.

In essence the administrator's role in developing a program for gifted/learning disabled children is rather like a gardener's. The seeds must be gathered, the soil prepared, the seeds planted, and a nurturing situation created. It is a tough job.

Chapter 20

Counseling Gifted/Learning Disabled Children

It would be helpful for teachers before reading this chapter to review Chapter 16 on the learning therapist. It is important to keep in mind that few teachers are trained as counselors and should not try to assume that role. However, throughout the course of every day, opportunities arise in the classroom to help children improve their self-esteem or assuage hurt egos.

One other aspect of teachers as counselors must be recognized and accepted by professional counselors, whether they be school counselors, school psychologists, clinical psychologists, or psychiatrists. The teacher has the opportunity to deal with problems immediately and in a relevant setting. These social and psychological dynamics usually are not present in an individual or group counseling session. Admittedly, these settings provide other types of opportunities to help the children. For their benefit, it is vital that all opportunities for assistance be seized.

TEACHER-THERAPIST COMMUNICATION

When a child is receiving therapy under any label outside of the classroom, the need for communication between that counselor/therapist and the teacher becomes paramount. The fundamental strategies and approaches to problems must be agreed upon and the procedures used by both adults must be in concert. They should hold face-to-face discussions in which specific anecdotes can be analyzed. (See Appendix 6-E on recordkeeping and daily anecdotal record sheets.)

If this type of concerted effort cannot be carried out, then the teacher must be sure to note in the child's record that the attempt was made. Many therapists prefer that their treatment be unaffected by information from other sources. It is their right to proceed in that fashion but the teacher must be covered.

A negative aspect if these adults do not work in concert is that it provides the child with an opportunity to play both ends against the middle. This is especially burdensome for the teacher since, without communication from the therapist, the child's responses, behaviors, etc., cannot be verified as legitimate. For example, a therapist may encourage a child to use physical retaliation to stand up to a bully. The teacher in the classroom is forced to deal with this retaliation as if it were aggression, using standard school procedures. Another approach might have been available if the teacher had been made aware of the therapist's goals.

Most children who have adjustment difficulties know only how to live within them. They tend not to be aware of more satisfactory modes of behavior. The role of counseling from whatever source should be fostering that perception. However, if infantile satisfaction can be obtained by pitting one adult against another: teacher-therapist, mother-father, sibling-sibling, etc., such children will do so. Uncoordinated responses and programs can only perpetuate the poor adjustment and its usual concomitant—poor learning.

PROBLEMS IN COUNSELING

Gifted/learning disabled children present a unique problem for counseling. In effect, they are multiexceptioned and, unfortunately for some, might be multi-handicapped. Other children with multiexceptionalities tend to have physical handicaps and cognitive disabilities. It is possible to have a blind/learning disabled child and many other dysfunctional combinations. In gifted/learning disabled children, both exceptionalities are nearly always cognitive and in many cases are recognized as polarities. It appears to be contradictory. It is this polarity that has led to the lack of understanding by the parents and teachers of these children and in the young people themselves. It also is the paradox that allows certain professionals to state that gifted/learning disabled children, by definition, cannot exist.

It is vital that the teacher operate with as much information as possible in dealing with these children. If possible, case history data should be obtained. It is important to know the home dynamics because these children all too frequently are the despair of their families. They are not and cannot be understood, yet they exist in the family and influence it, often profoundly.

Family data are important since such information could influence a teacher's reaction to a child or situation. Children who come from a laissez-faire household must be looked on differently from those in a home affected by academic or economic compulsion.

Understanding the Problem

The first step in teacher counseling of gifted/learning disabled children is an understanding of the problem they face. In most cases they have been told repeatedly that they are bright yet then are accused of laziness or indifference. The resolution of this paradox often is beyond the maturity or perception of most of these children. Therefore, the teacher's program must begin with basic education.

On the basis of their intelligence test scores, children can be shown what a percentile rating is and where in such a rating they stand. The teacher could ask, "If we lined up a hundred children your age from the brightest to the dullest, where do you think you would fit?" In most cases gifted/learning disabled children rate themselves very low on this scale yet often add, "People say I'm brighter." These children must be made aware of this giftedness and begin to accept it.

The Learning Disability Concept

The concept of learning disability also must be understood and discussed with these pupils. However, the teacher must be sure they understand that remedial and adaptive procedures are available to deal with the disability. Too frequently, children accept the disability and turn it into a handicap that they suffer through forever. Hope must always be available with help.

It should be on the basis of these two understandings that the explanation for changes in programming, instructional techniques, books, etc., is based. It is important for these children to begin to verbalize the reasons for certain procedures. Techniques such as the modified Fernald Procedure, which tends to be a slow process initially, have to be accepted as a way of learning rather than faster procedures that produce little or no real learning. Adaptive procedures that are effective must be accepted as legitimate means for turning frustration into success.

SOME CAUTIONS ESSENTIAL

Caution must be used when developing the understanding of giftedness and learning disability. In many instances there have been negative outcomes because reality has not been kept in the forefront of the children's perceptions. Immaturity is a trait easily observable in the gifted/learning disabled. These understandings can feed into this immaturity if permitted to do so. Children begin to use their exceptionalities for excuses. "I didn't do it because it was too easy for me," or "I couldn't do it because of my disability," or "You do know I am dyslexic, don't you?" become avoidance techniques for distasteful yet necessary behaviors.

In this situation, the teacher can move in at least two directions, based on the child's background. If the pupil has been hurt by failure, abrupt confrontation seldom avails anything. A better approach might be, "I know that you've tried things before and they didn't work so you need to say that not to get hurt. But I know you can do the things I asked, if you try. Would I ask you to do something if I thought you couldn't do it?"

The learning therapist section suggested that the teacher for a while has to become the child's superego. This is just such a situation. The idea of accepting the "rightness" of the request is transferred, at least for a while, from being the child's responsibility to being the teacher's. In many cases with gifted children, positive changes in this adjustment mechanism do not come quickly or easily. These children have lost their sense of confidence in self.

On the other hand, some may use these excuses for nearly infantile reasons. The pleasure-pain principle was never established. These kinds of children usually come from families that allowed them to excuse themselves from everything requiring emotional growth and control and in many cases to become tyrants. They get to feel omnipotent and accountable only to themselves.

The teacher in such a situation may have to take on a confrontation role. It may be necessary to say, "If it is so easy, do it for me and prove yourself right," or "So what if you are dyslexic, does that mean you can do anything you want to do to anybody at any time?" This also is the time to use the group as a focal point of reference. This highlights again the point made throughout this text: homogeneity of intelligence is needed in grouping this type of disabled child. The teacher might respond to the use of the handicapping level as an excuse with "I don't understand that. Many of the children in this group have been called dyslexic yet they seem to be doing things. How are you different from them?"

Whenever a confrontation approach is used, it is important that the child does not interpret the action as punitive. In such situations, it is important for the teacher to get as near eye level as possible, maintain eye contact, and keep the comments personal. It will only cause further hurt if the group is used as a means of shaming or disgracing the child. There is a very fine line that must be walked in this situation. The pupil must understand, especially because of the teacher's past behaviors, that this is a supportive technique.

During this discussion the child could be asked to analyze why the teacher is behaving in that fashion. It is important for the particular pupil and for all in the group that the teacher's behavior is planned and, if observed, changes from child to child.

This particular concept is crucial in teacher counseling. The children should know that they are all different and unique and therefore are not always treated the same. Neglect of this point often causes programs to fail in all educational settings. In certain situations, everyone is treated the same, with the same demands and privileges. However, in certain other respects, different children are treated differently. This point should be made as early as possible in the program. It should be stated to the group that this is the teacher's policy and its rationale should be explained. Making the statement clearly and early eliminates concern about favoritism and indifference. This concern of children with problems in adjustment can be so pervasive that nearly all of their energies are directed to it and thus are diverted from learning. As so often happens, the educational plan then is considered inadequate or inappropriate when in effect it never penetrated the child's comprehension.

FAILURE OR LACK OF SUCCESS

There is a point in the relationship between a student with problems and the teacher that is unique. This is the point of failure or perceived lack of success. Most gifted/learning disabled children have not enjoyed success commensurate with their abilities. In most cases this has been made very obvious to them. Some of them with good support from home and professional personnel enter remedial programs with hope for success. Others, even with the same support, start the program knowing they will fail.

Both groups can be found in remedial classrooms. Both groups have to encounter the phenomenon that education is based on—failure or lack of knowledge. Well-adjusted children see nothing wrong in error or ignorance and readily accept help. Many learning disabled children, especially those with excellent basic intelligence, view failure as the confirmation of their fundamental stupidity or as adult deceit. For teachers in these situations the counseling role is theirs alone. Therapists and counselors are not involved when a child errs or is unable to deal with an academic task.

For both types, this problem should be dealt with early, and preferably in a group situation so no child can feel singled out or stigmatized. The teacher must have at hand evidence of past successes but, most importantly, documented evidence of progress to reassure the hopeful child. When the child feels learning is hopeless, the same basic need for data is necessary but the evidence should be narrowed to those successes because such pupils often are overwhelmed by the use of progress data. They find that the idea of continuous progress seems unsustainable; this may well lead to a total halt in effort. They express the idea, "What's the use, I've got too far to go." The teacher in a counseling role must be extremely careful not to foster that attitude.

There also should be a wariness about dealing with success. (See Chapter 16 on the teacher as learning therapist.) The teacher must be aware that for many children, success brings with it failure. Quite simply, as stated by one child, "If I get this done, you're going to give me something harder." This is a statement not lacking perception. Too many teachers do not anticipate this possibility and in their enthusiasm at seeing progress forget that the child may view education as a never-ending process. Most adults know that that is true and tend to relish the idea. However, children—especially those who have found education painful and degrading—may not feel the same way.

The use of praise should be handled as carefully as reproach. As noted in the learning therapist segment, children who still need the teacher as a superego usually cannot handle praise. When this praise is elaborated into expected control and learning, these children seem only able to revert to past negative behavior or failure as if to prove that they are incapable of sustaining themselves. From an adjustment view, they probably are right.

THE ROLE OF RESPONSIBILITIES

During these interpersonal relationships between the individual child and the teacher, the latter needs to have enough ego to assume responsibilities and even blame for factors for which the instructor is not truly accountable. However, it is an important aspect of the role of teacher as counselor. When things have not gone right or well, the child should be given an indication that the teacher takes responsibility: "I guess I didn't understand how you would feel about that. How could I have done it differently so you wouldn't get upset?" or "I guess I asked you to do too much. How much do you think you could have done?"

However, the teacher never should assume the role of being the cause of the problem if the child is capable of correct behavior of whatever nature but simply has chosen not to conform or mature. At that point, confrontation may be the proper approach. If the child is truly unable to handle the tasks, mutual understanding must be redeveloped. To make progress, more limited types and degrees of responsibility should be tried, as suggested in the learning therapist chapter.

This limiting of tasks, if at all possible, should evolve out of the questions the teacher asks the child: "How could I have done it better . . . ," or "How much do you think you could have done?" This type of approach gives the child the reassurance that someone will listen and try to comply. It is a minor testimony of faith in the child as a reasonable human being.

When it appears that the pupil is capable of more self-direction, the teacher should suggest small increases in responsibilities or learning, making sure the child understands that positive support will be available no matter what the youngster's decision.

PROBLEM CHILD: THE ATTENTION SEEKER

There is another type that can be found in all classrooms yet presents a particular problem in a learning disabilities class: the attention-seeking child, who can be one of the most difficult to deal with therapeutically. This child often is labeled attention getting, which implies the pupil was successful in obtaining what was sought.

Attention-seeking in itself demonstrates a need. In most cases the need is for self-esteem or sense of self-worth or love. These children try to use their behavior to wrest these attributes from others. Their primary need is attention and they often will pay a severe price for it.

Attention and New Needs

The problem with learning disabled children, especially bright ones, is that in many cases they have had attention. They did not recognize it since it was in the form of testing, remedial programs, special classes, etc. Their problem is compounded since in most cases the attention has not worked. They still feel worthless and useless. A caution must be noted here. Some children feel that way because of traumatic factors in early life. They should be helped at the fundamental level of development by trained psychotherapists with attending support from the teacher.

The first task the teacher as counselor must face is to develop in attention-seeking children an understanding of their behavior. Punishment will not do, as is discussed later. This is a time for direct, intimate conversation in which the beginning levels of introspection can be put in place. Simply requesting that the child try to enumerate some reasons for the behavior is a starting point. At times the teacher can make simple suggestions about possibilities that have been observed. The daily record sheet with its anecdotes can prove useful.

The second aspect for discussion should be an understanding about negative and positive attention. It is amazing the number of very intelligent children who are unable to discern this difference. The teacher should ask for some actions that the child could have used to get positive, rather than negative, attention. The concept of laugh with, rather than laugh at, is useful.

Punishment Counterproductive

These children's lack of understanding of the negative/positive attention concept is the reason that punishment as a technique often is counterproductive. When they are punished, they receive attention and in some cases all the attention of their classmates as well as of the teacher. This negative reinforcement of useless, disruptive behavior can become quite addictive to many children.

As early as possible, punishment should be moved from the hands of the teacher to the hands of the child. The concept that "you punish yourself" should be promoted. Rules should be set down so that children know the consequences, positively and negatively, of their behavior: "If you get your work finished, you would have time to play a game with your friend, or use the computer," or "If that follow-up isn't done, how are you going to get to use the computer?"

Every attempt should be made in these situations with attention-seekers for the teacher to be an arbitrator between the child and the behavior. The judge and jury roles too often play into the hands of the attention-seeking child. It is not easy for the teacher to maintain controls in these situations but it must be kept in mind that if they are not maintained, the problem only becomes worse and undoubtedly is prolonged.

Positive Attention

Examples of positive attention in many cases must be verbalized. A child can simply be asked to state some positive behaviors. In most cases it is better to start with social behaviors that have to do with individual or group acceptance. Simple techniques for positive entry into groups may have to be discussed. How does one get into a group game or group conversation? Food sharing, swapping, etc., can be helpful in moderation. These techniques must be monitored and discussed since in these situations attention-seekers often tend to go overboard and bring themselves into ridicule, which is another form of negative attention.

In some cases, frank discussions about hair, clothes, hygiene, etc., may have to be initiated since these factors can get negative attention. Older girls often become sexually provocative for no reason other than the need for attention. In these situations frank, honest observations by the teacher concerning possible reasons for the behaviors are pertinent and suggestions for changes are appropriate.

Academic negation can be handled more easily if strides have been made in the social aspects. The teacher should let the children know that making honest errors is acceptable but that deliberately failing, in order to command attention, will not be tolerated. When appropriate, the teacher should share the joy of success with the individual and sometimes with the group. Recognition from a teacher is important for most children.

The teacher in the counselor's role should conduct certain procedural aspects on an individual basis. However, a number of procedures can be handled in the group setting. The initial group effort has been discussed already; everyone is not always treated the same in all things.

A second important facet of the group procedure is the development of the nature of its members. There is a valid reason to keep their giftedness in front of them. They must accept their abilities and learn to live with the positive and negative aspects. Factors suggested for this concept with individuals are equally as valid for groups. The use of percentiles and line graphs can become concrete enough to be used as referents when an individual child begins to have troubles.

PLANNING ON THEIR OWN

All learning disabled children should be given time for daily initial planning and daily final evaluation. The initial planning phase is important as it should provide them with the structure they usually need. It also can be a time of sharing. However, caution must be observed in this respect.

Sharing is a particularly upsetting activity for many attention-seeking children. It can provide an opportunity for the "clowns" in the group to make fools of themselves and get the appropriate negative attention. For others, it can become a time to demonstrate their inabilities or handicaps. In some instances these children will do and say things to bring ridicule on themselves, which again provides the desired negative attention.

In both of these situations the teacher's counseling role begins before the activity. A deliberate check of a proposed sharing presentation should be made and anything inappropriate rejected, with an explanation. Suggestions for other types or degrees of participation are legitimate as well as a direct personal evaluation of the reason behind the inappropriate behavior. One child who was fanatical about dinosaurs made a fool of himself by labeling them wrong, forgetting their names, etc., and admitted doing so because "Nobody even thinks this is important so at least they laughed at me."

Show-and-tell activities at any time of the day are apt to produce problems, even if only of a subtle nature. When they are used with children having adjustment difficulties, they can be disruptive to the program and deleterious to certain pupils. Teacher monitoring is demanded. In some instances children have participated in these activities using articles that were dangerous, inappropriate, or even pornographic because the teacher did not monitor what was to be done.

The daily final evaluation in the group of the group is a crucial activity for gifted/learning disabled children. It is here that some of the best opportunities are provided for the introduction of flexibility and adaptability. Answers can be elicited from the group concerning other methods of doing things, other types of procedures, and other ways of thinking or viewing things. Too frequently, this very important element in the instructional program is excluded completely. When appropriate, during this activity, individuals can be called on to provide information, suggest courses of action, etc., and obtain positive attention.

It usually is risky for anyone not professionally trained in counseling or therapy to try to use group practices as a direct medium for individual guidance activities involving group dynamics. It is more appropriate to use the groups as a supplement to the development of the individual on a one-to-one basis. With gifted/learning disabled children, group activities do not appear to be the best approach, as suggested above.

In certain situations, especially in private schools for children with problems, professional counseling or psychotherapy is provided during the academic day. This causes problems for the teacher as counselor. Communication between the counselor/therapist and the teacher is mandatory. There is really no other satisfactory procedure if the children are to make progress academically as well as psychologically.

The type of therapy being used by the child's personal therapist also can be a problem. In most cases children returning from individual "talk" therapy might be a little morose or too exuberant but usually not to such a degree that the academic program is completely disrupted. The same cannot be said in many cases where the children are in group or play therapy. They frequently return to the classroom quite hyperactive and try to extend group therapy to the class or instructional group. They seem unable to recognize the differences in the two situations. This is another example of the flexibility and adaptability problem.

Play therapy causes the same type of behavior. Children who have sublimated or denied feelings for years find an acceptable outlet in play therapy and become almost intoxicated with the emotional release. When returning to the classroom they are reluctant to assume a more placid or conforming role. These behaviors can disrupt the educational program to such a degree that the teacher has to abandon all plans while attempting to restore an academic environment. The children must always be faced with the concept that their teacher is there first of all as an educator.

METHODS OF COPING

A number of ways exist to meet this problem. As was suggested earlier, teacher-therapist communication is a must. As another method, group and play therapy sessions should be scheduled so that afterward the children are through for the day or are going to lunch or to any activity other than receiving instruction. If these arrangements are not possible, the teacher must request that the therapist finish the session by reinstating some controls. The teacher should schedule the children so that the block of time in their programs to which they are returning is either independent activities or independent reading. (See Chapter 18 on classroom management procedures.) They should not be scheduled into instruction or follow-up activities.

Finally, there is an aspect of the counselor role that is particularly pertinent to the teacher. If things have gone well in the teacher-children personal relationships, an unsettling condition must be faced. Eventually, the relationships must be terminated. Eventually all contacts will cease and some piece of each individual's ego will be lost. Most teachers and nearly all the children either forget or ignore this finality. But it does occur—every year. It is important that the teachers of learning disabled children of all types keep this in mind because when the termination becomes apparent to the pupils, a rather specific phenomenon emerges: separation anxiety.

Teacher-child personal relationships often become quite close. Deep fears, longings, and loves have been shared. A confidence has been developed that for some children may have been the first and possibly the only time they have ever known that trait. Yet this relationship must end. School will close; summer vacation will begin.

To protect themselves, some pupils may revert to former childish behaviors. Others actually will show losses in skills and abilities. Still others may become sullen and even rude toward the teacher. All of these behaviors seem to be a defense that says, "See, you are not that important to me. You didn't help me. I don't need you." If individuals really are so unimportant, they cannot be missed too much; the hurt cannot be too bad.

Teachers, when dealing with this separation anxiety, must be sure to recognize what it is and not allow it to impinge negatively on their own feelings. It is important to help children deal with it individually, not in group activities, since their reactions will be unique. The teachers should provide evidences of continuing care by suggesting meetings during the coming year, exchanges of cards over the summer, and sharing of information if meetings are not possible. Teachers also must be willing to verbalize their feelings when they are genuine. They should let the children know that having warm, positive feelings for other people is a fine, human trait and nothing to be ashamed of; caring and loving are what life is really about. For many gifted/learning disabled children these two relationships seem to be distorted, whether in fact or in faulty perception; which of these is unimportant, since the children believe it and operate with it. During the period of separation anxiety, the teacher's thoughtfulness in handling this reaction can make a significant positive change in a child's emotional outlook.

TOUCHING: PLUSES AND MINUSES

Throughout this chapter, the teacher's role as therapist has been discussed in such a way as to suggest language and role modeling are the only two techniques available. There is another fundamental, very human counseling technique that must be handled carefully. However, it can be useful and necessary. The technique is touching as a fundamental source of human contact.

Children appear to like to be touched. However, because of some particular problems, many resist touching and, when this resistance is analyzed, it is found to be based on fear. Since touching is so intimate, relationships involved with touching tend to be strong. If something happens that makes the relationship disappear or become hurtful, children often react negatively to touch.

Initially, it is easy to gauge whether there is a problem by simply placing a hand on a shoulder. If the child flinches or pulls away, a problem is apparent. At a more opportune time later, the child can be asked outright the reason for pulling away. The answer usually is based on disliking it. If the child is asked why, there usually is no initial response. Later, when introspection has developed, reasons are usually forthcoming.

Touching is a valuable tool for teachers. A firm squeeze of an arm can indicate "I want you to control yourself." A gentler squeeze of a shoulder can mean "Well done." Two foreheads against each other can mean "I sympathize with you." The touching codes that develop with children with problems often become the most important tool of the teacher as counselor.

As with all techniques, touching is no panacea. Certain children never get over their negative reactions to touching unless psychotherapy is successful. Others overreact and need to have limits established. Some are "clinging vines" who need to learn to free themselves from the need of too much support. This can be handled by discussing when such behaviors are inappropriate and why, and then when they can be appropriate.

Still other children may use touching as a means of infantile gratification. Some actually will maul a teacher or other children, using their hands in a totally inappropriate fashion; little boys may investigate older females out of curiosity. Too often these behaviors are considered cute. The fundamental approach to this problem in the classroom appears to be the setting of limits. These limits must be understood by the child and by the group, and the teacher as counselor must demand adherence. This also is the time that a recommendation for private therapy can be made through appropriate channels.

SUMMARY

The role of the teacher as counselor might be summed up in a simple statement: the teacher must care about the child as a human being, not just as a student. Any situation in which an individual's own needs are intertwined with those of others always carries with it the chance for hurt. The teacher as the adult and better adjusted member of the pair must be willing to roll with the punches and see through the reasons for the behavior. The returns for caring are enormous.

Chapter 21

Counseling Parents

When dealing with parents of gifted/learning disabled children, it is important to keep in mind what role the teacher as counselor may take and what role is to be avoided. In most instances the teacher's role must be confined to factors that influence the educational program. Overall household dynamics that are destructive or disruptive to overall family life must be left to a specialist in family counseling or family therapy.

ACQUIRING INFORMATION

One of the first problems the teacher faces in the counselor role is obtaining useful information. A major hurdle in helping many learning disabled children is how the family views the etiology of the problem. One of two points of view usually is quite evident. (See Chapter 16 on the teacher as learning therapist.) One view is that the child carried adjustment problems to school and because of them failure ensued. The other view is that the school failed to provide an adequate, suitable program and the child therefore developed adjustment difficulties because of academic failure.

Most parents prefer the second idea because it does free them from the responsibility of causation. However, by the time a child is placed in a program for exceptional pupils the dichotomy has little practical significance. Further discussions can be of little value. The here and now must be discussed and understood.

If a teacher is to provide counseling help to parents under the restrictions noted above, confidence based on impartiality must be established. It must be evident to the parents that the teacher is genuinely interested in the child's welfare and is willing to invest time and energy with them as well as the pupil. This accepting relationship is so important that if it does not exist, the teacher's role in this respect should not be attempted.

When a relationship has been developed, the concept of confidentiality between teacher and parents must be accepted by both parties. This means that in certain cases the teacher must not share information with anyone unless the parents agree. This concept must be discussed bluntly. The need to share information is important and the parents need to respect the teacher's judgment in such matters. The recognition of genuine caring is helpful in establishing these guidelines.

Probably the most important concept that parents and teacher must agree upon is that the child will not be allowed to play both ends against the middle. What the child says or reports to either party should be checked by the other side before any action is taken. In this way the upsurge of emotionality that parents display so often can be tempered. The teacher's cultivation of this type of delayed response has an important carryover in the parent-child relationship.

The cultivation of the delayed response in the parents is another early goal in this counseling. It usually is carried out best by discussions with the parents about alternatives. It is important that thinking about alternatives is stimulated first before an attempt is made to have the process put into action. Simple questions such as, "What other things could you do in this situation?" or "How many things do you think could have caused the child to do that?" or "Really, how did that behavior affect you? Why?" can be a foundation in changing parent attitudes and behaviors.

In many cases this can be done best in a group situation, using examples or simulations. Initially, parents can sit silent, shielded by anonymity, but once the interactions begin, they tend to become quite specific about their children and themselves. The sharing of the problems is important but the value of other alternative behaviors or different perceptions cannot be overestimated.

ORDERLY COMMUNICATION VITAL

The teacher's goals and planning must be shared with the parents and understanding of these elements must be developed. The first of these involves orderly communication. This is the area in which the weekly report form discussed in Chapter 18 (on classroom management procedures) is so important. Parents must be helped to understand what the report contains and what the information means. They must be helped in using the information. They also must understand that there is a system to be used. The report is given to the child and initialled daily by the teacher. The report goes home with both teacher and child comments. The parents discuss the report with the child. Both positive and negative aspects receive attention and appropriate courses of action can be followed. A follow-up conference can be arranged when appropriate. The ability to see and use alternatives (as mentioned earlier in this segment) and the need to weigh different courses of actions make the use of the weekly report an effective instrument.

At this time a new form of dynamics can be introduced if required. The responsibility for the weekly report is from child to parent, not teacher to parent. If a parent does not receive the report and calls, the teacher should reply, "I sent it home with your youngster, you'd better check and see why it did not get home," or, if it was not returned to the teacher, the answer should be "You had better find out why your youngster did not return the report to me."

It is mandatory that this responsibility be kept with the parents. Under no circumstances should the teacher assume this role.

However, these concepts must be tempered by the reality that some parents do not care and therefore their roles are minimal or disruptive. Other parents may not be able to understand the reasoning behind the plan of action. One mother, after receiving what appeared to be a very lucid presentation of the child's problems and possible courses of action, announced on leaving the conference, "Don't worry, as soon as I get home I'll give him a good beating."

In situations where there is parental indifference, the teacher as counselor must focus on the development in the child of a self-caring, self-respecting attitude. In the case of little or no parental understanding, concentration again must be directed toward the child. With the parents, it is helpful to develop a plan of action that is almost ordained: "If this happens, I want you to do this for or to the child." As much as routines can be detrimental to the children's progress, in this circumstance a routine can become supportive and developmental even if the parents do not clearly understand the rationale behind it. In such a situation, alternatives must be limited in number and rather circumscribed in application.

These courses of action usually are helpful for gifted/learning disabled children. Parents who may be bewildered by the "bright dumb child" need not try to reason out the dilemma. The child begins to be dealt with consistently and demands on adaptability are reduced. The adaptable child usually can cope with parental ups and downs if the swings are not too violent. Unfortunately, gifted/learning disabled children often disintegrate in that type of environment if it is at all severe. The more the teacher as counselor can help the parents behave systematically and consistently, the better the chances of success in academic areas.

THE CONCEPT OF GIFTEDNESS

The teacher as counselor must carry out another communications task especially for the parents of gifted/learning disabled children: educate them as to the concept of giftedness. This concept often is too difficult for professionals to accept, so parents need guidance. It is often hard to accept a child who is failing academically as very intelligent. The concept must be explained to the parents and if possible demonstrated by examples of such behavior, e.g., excellent problem perceptions, discovering alternative solutions, etc. Learning disability must be handled in the same manner. These parents need to be able to relate the polarities of their children's behavior to understandable concepts, not just to labels. The traits of these children (listed in Chapter 2 on characteristics and traits) should be dealt with. However, the teacher should try to develop these traits not as a totality but one by one. Parental observation of specific behaviors, and the sharing of those observations, should be encouraged. This aspect of the counseling procedure is better done in a group whenever feasible. The value of sharing noted earlier is just as important here.

These understandings should provide an opportunity to foster a concept that is truly necessary if the total program is to be successful. Many of these parents, as noted, blame the school for the child's failure and resent anything that appears to discriminate against their offspring. Yet it has been advocated here that teachers must discriminate in the way they treat a child based on individual uniqueness. Everyone should not be treated the same. Parents must be informed of this concept and the reasons for the teacher's action. If parents truly believe that the treatment is based on caring and they have been informed how different children need to be treated differently because of their uniqueness, they can accept this varied approach to instruction and deportment demands.

This also is an opportune time to develop the idea of learning plateaus. Many parents have difficulty accepting learning as growth in spurts. They all recognize it in the children's physical growth but often fail to transfer the idea to cognitive development. If a weekly report system is to be effective, parents must accept this understanding.

PARENTAL BEHAVIOR: HELP AND CAUTION

It is in the area of parental behavior in the home that the teacher as counselor must be fully alert. If what the teacher is going to suggest cannot or will not be accepted by the parents, the instructor should attempt to have them obtain professional help but should not become involved in dynamics that require higher level understandings and, most importantly, much different procedures. No teacher should feel incompetent if family relationships do not improve. In fact, in certain situations, improvement may not be possible. Teachers must remember that in some instances children are institutionalized or put into foster homes because of this parental problem.

Certain changes in family reactions can be suggested. The most important area is the handling of the child's attention-getting behaviors. Parents must be helped to understand positive and negative attention. As was noted in the section on counseling children, some pupils do not and cannot differentiate negative from positive attention. They only recognize attention. The same thing also can be said of some parents. The teacher should develop this concept in the group sessions, then encourage parents to state personal examples of it. The group should be given some examples or simulations and should classify the behaviors. The teacher can ask for suggestions on how to develop positive attention techniques. If possible the teacher should make a few or no suggestions if the group offers good ideas and should try to help it become more self-sustaining through group interaction. In cases where faulty ideas are presented, the teacher should not be reluctant to intrude with ideas. One of the goals of the counselor program is the development of the teacher as an authority figure in certain areas who can be supportive of the child and the family.

The role of praise and punishment should be natural components in the attention-seeking area. Too frequently a reaction sets in as parents become aware of their role in a child's academic development. The child becomes "family fragile." This means that the demands, responsibilities, and punishment of the family are eliminated. The child is developing the opportunity to become the family tyrant. In the group sessions it is as important to confront the parents with reality as it is to do so with the child in academic activities.

Parents should be encouraged to increase the child's family responsibilities as progress continues. They should make demands that are reasonable and in line with those on other children as a reality of life. These responsibilities and demands should not appear to be punitive but as part of family living. The concept that, "since you were bad, you have to do the dishes tonight," should not be used. Dishwashing is a family chore for which all members should be responsible in some degree.

A more difficult area in helping parents involves punishment. Parents should take the same attitude as teachers in this area: children punish themselves. If things are done right or behavior is satisfactory, no punishment ensues. However, if either or both of these are not true, then punishment is the outcome.

It is in this area that the most work in parent counseling must be done. The "children punishing themselves" concept can be effective only in an orderly household. Rules, regulations, and responsibilities must be understood clearly and delineated for all the members. Alternative punishments also must be clearly understood. The parents must have developed a talking relationship with the child. In such a situation, they must transfer the delayed response reaction and use of alternatives to their dealings with the children. This pattern of response is not too difficult to develop if home and school work on it together.

However, the emphasis in these situations must always return to the opportunities for positive attention and parents should help children consider the effects of alternatives: "You see, if you had done the work this afternoon when you had time, you could be watching that TV show right now." The responsibility is being given to the child. It is important, however, for all adults dealing with children who are trying to mature that these elders do not let the young people go completely unaided. Simple suggestions of present behaviors that will result in unfavorable consequences can help a child pursue a happier course of action. The weighing of alternatives is a developmental task, also.

In attention-getting behavior areas, the foundation of understanding usually can be developed in a group situation. However, many of the specific techniques for parents to use in dealing with this area should be proposed in parent conferences. These techniques were enumerated in Chapter 20. Families are so diverse in so many important aspects that individual approaches are more appropriate. Confidentiality is important in many cases when this aspect of child control is being carried out.

Finally, parents' reactions often involve an underlying element of guilt. Sometimes they verbalize this openly; in other instances, they recognize it only as it is projected onto others. For many parents, it is a terrible burden. They feel that the fact that the child possibly was unplanned or unwanted is responsible for the problem. A working mother or too-busy father may develop guilt because they perceive a lack of positive attention toward the child.

A teacher can be helpful in assisting parents to deal with their feelings of guilt. The first and best response is positive: "Did you do what you thought was best for the child? Then what else could you do?" or "Once the baby was born, did you accept the child? Have you tried to do your best for the child?"

The same basic approach can be helpful in addressing etiology. The teacher should analyze whether the parents have recognized that the elements that cause disability are numerous and exist in all realms of a child's life. The use of a group forum is a valuable tool in dealing with this problem. However, the initial work often is best done in individual sessions. Group sessions tend to be useful for broadening the concept rather than for initiating the realization.

Once parents realize that guilt is a normal reaction, the next step is for them to accept the here and now—what should be done, at what time, and at what place. The past and all the "might have beens" have to be relegated to a minor position. The overall planning and coordination of adult behavior must become the emphasis of the teacher's counseling. Positive changes in the child brought about by thoughtful handling, especially from the parents, usually assuage much guilt.

SUMMARY

It must be restated that the teacher as counselor role for families requires an initial high level of perception. If the child or the family is emotionally disturbed, the instructor should function as a teacher and obtain guidance from a professional counselor or therapist. If the family dynamics are such that academic growth is curtailed, the teacher should inform the appropriate superior of this opinion as protection against unrealistic criticism.

There are rewards for helping parents manage their children better. There are rewards in personal satisfaction and in the children's progress. There also are problems if objectivity is lost. When this happens, child, family, and teacher all suffer.

Index

About the Author

Paul R. Daniels is professor of education in the evening college and summer session of The Johns Hopkins University in Baltimore, Maryland. He received his doctorate in the psychology of reading from Temple University in Philadelphia, Pennsylvania. Dr. Daniels began working with severely retarded readers in the laboratory school of the reading clinic of Temple University as a teacher and finally the supervisor of the school. After 17 years, Dr. Daniels became an associate professor of reading at Loyola College in Baltimore, Maryland. He then became instructional consultant and coordinating supervisor of reading in Prince George's County, Maryland. For the last ten years, Dr. Daniels has been in charge of the graduate program in reading at Johns Hopkins. For more than three decades, Dr. Daniels worked with children from public and private schools, faculties, and other clinical support personnel. He is past president of the Disabled Reader Special Interest Group of the International Reading Association and president elect of the Multidisciplinary Academy of Clinical Education.